KRISTINA HARRIS

VINTAGE
Fashions
FOR
Women
1920s - 1940s

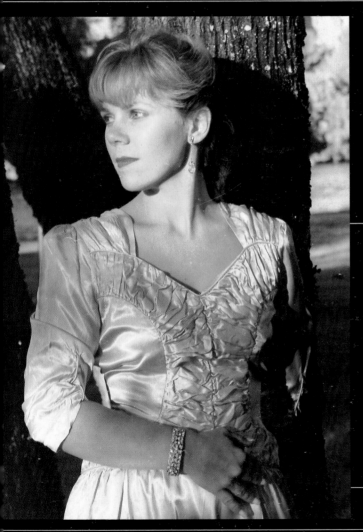

WITH VALUES

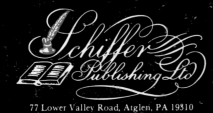

Schiffer Publishing Ltd

77 Lower Valley Road, Atglen, PA 19310

Library of Congress Cataloging-in-Publication Data

Harris, Kristina.
    Vintage fashions for women 1920s-1940s / Kristina Harris.
        p. cm.
    Includes bibliographical references and index.
    ISBN 0-88740-986-5 (pbk.)
    1. Costume--United States--History--2oth century. 2. Fashion--United
States--History--20th century. 3. Vintage clothing--United States. I. Title.
    GT615.H37 1996
    391'.2'09730904--dc20   96-2517
                                                                   CIP

Printed in Hong Kong
ISBN 0-88740-986-5

Published by Schiffer Publishing Ltd.
77 Lower Valley Road
Atglen, PA 19310
Please write for a free catalog.
This book may be purchased from the publisher.
Please include $2.95 for shipping.
Try your bookstore first.

440 6910

ACKNOWLEDGMENTS

No one person makes any book reality; it takes the energy and enthusiasm of a great many people, and I thank everyone who has made this book possible.

Thank you to the board of The Very Little Theatre in Eugene, Oregon for allowing me access to their collection. Who would have ever imagined a little community theatre in Oregon would have such a marvelous collection of antique and vintage fashions! Special thanks is also extended to Lucy Sullivan (matchmaker and marketing agent extraordinaire), who took the time to help me explore the collection, and never seemed surprised when I uncovered another beaded dress or pair of shoes from the costume shop's nooks and crannies. *And* she test–modeled all the hats for me!

Thanks is also extended to Darwin Sullivan, who kindly took the time to uncover an authentic World War II Navy uniform for me.

Others kindly lent me pieces from their collections so that I could photograph them for this book. For trusting me with your treasures, I thank enthusiasts Sharon Jones and Dorothy Wright, and enthusiasts/dealers Priscilla Washco of Persona Vintage Clothing in Astoria, Oregon and Marlene J. Minnich of Marianine's Vintage Chic in Lehighton, Pennsylvania.

For allowing me to shoot the photographs on location, my appreciation is extended to Myra Plant of the Campbell House Inn in Eugene, Oregon; Marjory Gossler of Gossler Farms Nursery in Springfield, Oregon; and Jan Alberg and the board of the historic Shelton-McMurphy-Johnson House in Eugene, Oregon.

My gratitude is also extended to the models, who (when they weren't busy ooh-ing and ahh-ing over the clothes, or asking me if they could take any of them home) put up admirably with too-tight screw-on earrings and uncomfortable shoes. Again, the book wouldn't have been the same without you! Thank you: Anna Kristine Crivello, Clinton McKay Crivello, Lisa Ann Crivello, Jocelyn Jones, Darcie Jones, Stephanie Jones, Alicia Lafayette, and Virginia Speckman.

And finally, a big thank you is due to my mother, who, as always, donated time, energy, and a helping hand.

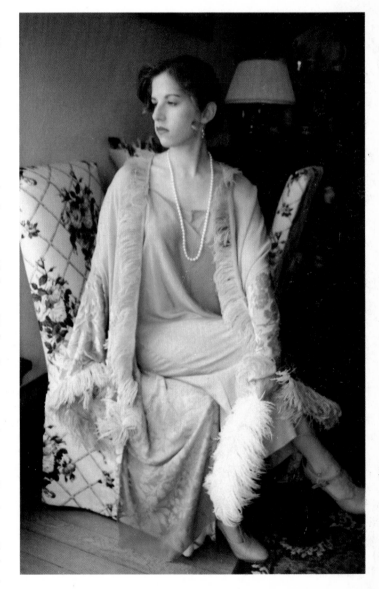

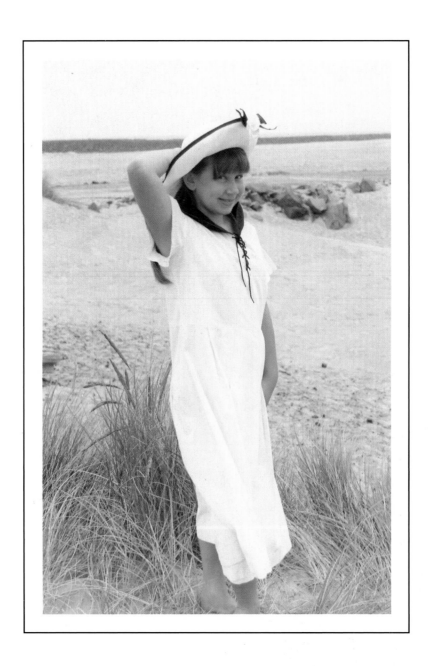

CONTENTS

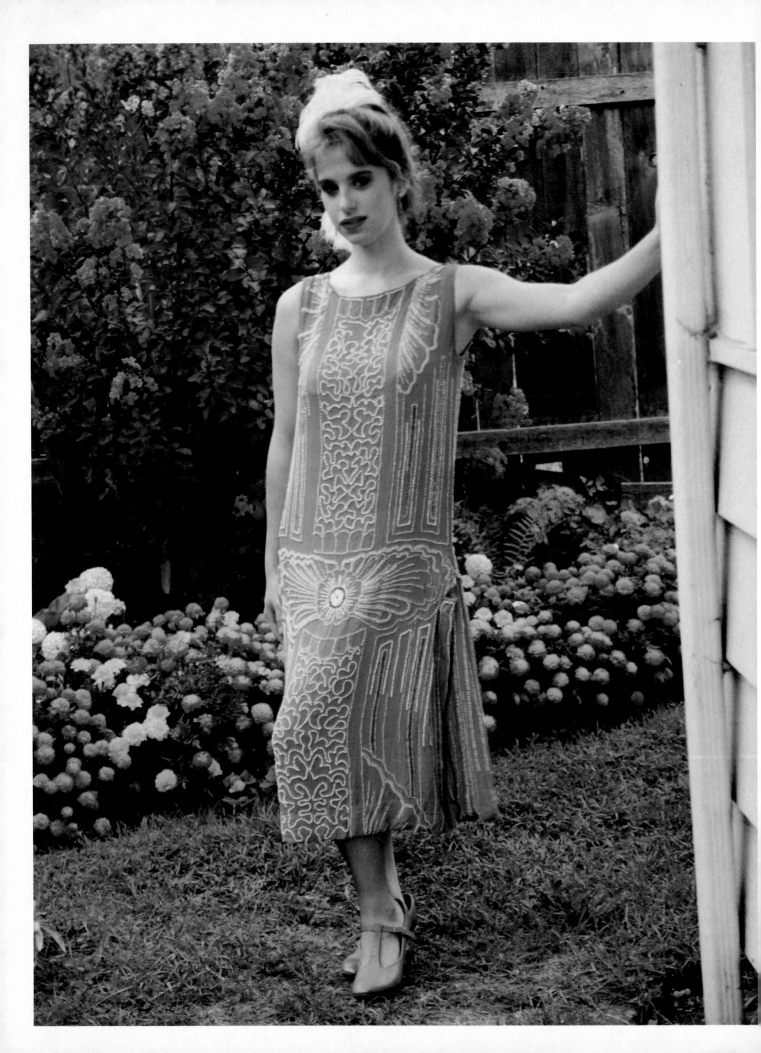

INTRODUCTION

In a carefully padded antique trunk which sits beside me lays a treasure. It is a fragile wisp of history: a breezy chiffon chemise–style flapper dress. Long, tubular, and with the tiniest of cap sleeves, it is the epitome of an era. Hundreds—possibly thousands—of clear bugle beads and tiny, white, round beads embellish the dress from its scooping neckline to its fat, handstitched hem. Straight from the hip, a wide, gaping eye with squiggly lines bursting from it stares at me, daring me to remember that there was a time when the esoteric appeal of King Tut's tomb was so universal that fashion took a moment to relish in it.

Peeking behind the textured exterior of the dress, skilled, double-stitched lines of thread reveal themselves beneath the weight of the tiny—but heavy—glass beads . . . Hand-finished seams lay flat and unobtrusive . . . Crisp little pleats—barely noticeable on the highly decorative exterior—appear, perfectly stitched.

But I can peer even further into the story of this little dress. Though once it may have been a favorite party dress of a 1920s woman, it somehow made its way into the costume department of Paramount Pictures. Perhaps it even originated there, since Paramount was already spreading the magic of movies by the 1920s. For decades the dress sat, largely unattended, in Paramount's vast costume department—until fairly recently, when a Roaring Twenties costume party was announced, and the dress was freed from its confines to be given to one of the party-goers.

For several years after, the dress was tucked away in a cardboard box, and pulled out whenever a costume party was announced—until the day I met that party-goer. Knowing my passion for clothes of the past, she kindly gave me the dress—now musty and wrinkled with age and use.

From the individual beauty or character of a 1920s dress, a sleek 1930s evening gown, or a refined 1940s suit, to the bits of history recoverable from each garment's past, right down to how and from whom you acquired the piece, the world of vintage fashions is all-consuming. For those who know the thrill of the hunt, the satisfaction and pride of finally finding a long-sought-after piece, the pure joy of studying and displaying a fashion collection, there is nothing else quite like it.

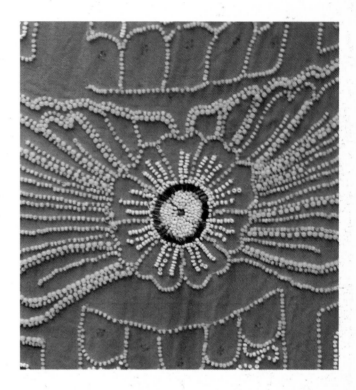

You know you have officially become a vintage fashion collector when you go out to shop for milk or aspirin, and find yourself inside vintage clothing and antique shops, surrounded by piles of veri–colored textiles, racks of musty clothes, and piles of yellowing sewing patterns, fashion plates, and magazines. It may start slowly—perhaps with a family heirloom. Still, slowly but surely, a fantastically feathered forties hat will find its way to your home . . . then you discover a "little black dress" from the thirties that you can't resist—it was such a steal!

There are still those who treasure only the very rare or expensive—Chanel accessories, Schiaparelli evening gowns—but many of today's collectors find it is the more "everyday" things of yesterday that are most intriguing. Designer garments have skyrocketed to unheard-of prices, leaving the average collector far, *far* behind. Still, collectors know that while couture designs may be whimsical and fantastic, they hardly represent what the average woman wore. With a new sense of understanding, the "everyday" woman is emerging—and, thankfully, there are still many fine examples of her wardrobe available for today's collector.

There is a wealth of fashion history books that deal almost exclusively with couture designs (which very often have little to do with what most women were wearing) and European war-years fashions. But there is a great void of information on ready-to-wear and other "average" American garments. I have tried to help fill this void, by picturing such garments and by offering up details about them. This book being a collectors' guide and not a tour of fashion history, I have limited the garments pictured to those that the average collector can obtain.

While it is certainly interesting to admire and collect couture designer wear, collectors should never let anyone tell them that non-couture designer clothing is less collectible. I think time will prove that the opposite is true. Museums, historians, and avid collectors have found that non-designer fashions tell them much more about most women of the nineteenth century—and I think they will soon discover the same is true for women of the twentieth century.

There is always another old dress lurking around the corner, waiting to be rescued. There's always another neglected forties evening gown, or Depression-era hat, or flapper-era bag hoping to find an owner who will be perceptive enough to see through decades of dust and stains and carefully nurture it back to something of its original self. These are the treasures of our mothers and grandmothers. They are the essence of the American woman—the first styles American women actually began to tailor to themselves, rather than just copying European garb. And like the little beaded dress that sits beside me, they are not treasures that are only attainable to the wealthy. As I hope this book proves, the joy of collecting and learning from the modes of the past is accessible to us all.

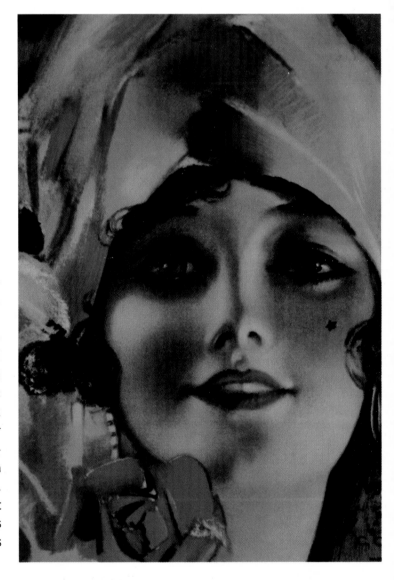

AUTHOR'S NOTE

Like many thoughtful people in the field, I believe in the conservation of clothing as artifacts. This a heated topic in the world of vintage clothing. Museum curators, researchers, and historians know that the wearing of vintage clothing leads to the destruction of historical artifacts. Yet I have chosen to photograph the garments in this book by modeling them not on mannequins, but on live persons.

If this seems contradictory to my assertion that fashions should be preserved, let me explain myself.

I believe that clothing, like any other artifact, is best appreciated if it is well presented. For example, we rarely see antique furniture presented in a museum under a glass case, solitary from other furniture and decor. And just as a Rococo settee seems less influential without a decorated room as its natural companion, so clothing somehow seems less adequate hung on a wall or set atop a mannequin.

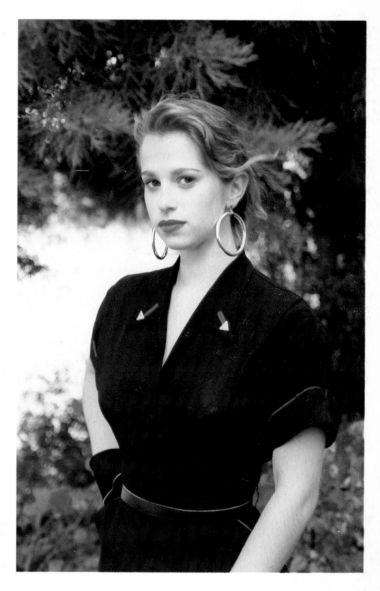

There is no better way to appreciate the value, craftsmanship, and beauty of vintage clothing than to view it as it was intended to be seen—on a live figure.

And for those like me, who are concerned that placing vintage fashions on live models can be hazardous to the clothing's health, let me ease your concerns. No article of clothing was worn by any model if it was in an extremely fragile state. All models were well educated about the fragile state of the garments being photographed. No surroundings were allowed to stain, rip, or harm the garments photographed in any way. Unlike a fashion show, our photo sessions allowed ample time for the models to get in and out of the garments with care. No garment was worn for more than a few minutes, and they were always carefully protected.

In fact, because the garments modeled for this book were worn only briefly, they were probably in less danger of harm than garments mounted onto mannequins and displayed for an exhibition.

Finally, for those who are reading this note and wondering what all this fuss is about, please be sure to read Chapter One for more information.

COLLECTING VINTAGE FASHIONS

The fashions created and worn from 1920 through the 1940s are uniquely intimate to collectors. These are the fashions our parents and grandparents (and perhaps our great-grandparents) wore. They are the styles we've become familiar with through our family scrapbooks; fashions permanently documented by sepia-toned photographs with pinked edges: the simple chemise-like dress and rolled hose your grandmother posed in beside the family roadster . . . the sleek, rhinestone-embellished evening dress modeled by your mother while she was still in her teens . . . the wide-shouldered wool suit your aunt wore to pose beside your uncle, while he was on furlough and in uniform. Though it may at first seem a strange thought, today's vintage clothing—those fashions from our family albums—are tomorrow's antique artifacts.

To Wear Or Not To Wear

Perhaps because vintage fashions are so "young" and familiar to us, many collectors want to wear them. Dressing up in the elegance of the past seems easy enough, since vintage clothing often fits in reasonably well with today's eclectic fashions. However, not only will vintage clothing rip and eventually fall to pieces if even slightly too small, but wearing vintage clothing usually destroys the collectibility and historical significance of the piece. Consider, for instance, how we treat other collectibles—like a porcelain teapot from, say, the early 1900s. Bought in an antique store, most of us would actually be afraid to use the pretty little item and would instead place it in a china cabinet or on a visible shelf for display. Yet, take a 1920s beaded dress bought at a vintage clothing store; many collectors would have no qualms about wearing it. Yet it is just as fragile as the porcelain teapot (even more so!). And surely the dress is a more important artifact.

Previous Page:
Though much of the "everyday" fashions of the 1930s are rare today, evening gowns from the period are readily available.

Only so many pieces of vintage clothing were ever created, and only a fraction of those have survived till today. Thinking of your collection in these terms, you'll quickly realize that proper care is essential.

To fulfill the natural urge to show off your collection, try exploring other options. How about displaying special pieces in your home, framed under ultra–violet glass or protected by archive-quality collector's display cases? (Just be certain to rotate your displays frequently, since light, heat, moisture, dust, and humidity are great destroyers of textiles.) Or perhaps you'd enjoy lending pieces from your collection to local museums or historic buildings for their rotating display?

If you still wish to actually *wear* vintage styles, you can dress in reproductions. These are readily available either ready-made or in pattern form, and are frequently advertised in vintage clothing related periodicals.

I recognize, however, that no matter how much any person or organization recommends otherwise, there will always be collectors who wear vintage clothing—so please allow me to offer some guidelines which may help lessen the harm this does. First and foremost, I would ask that you never alter any garment. This destroys both the monetary and historical value of the piece. The one exception to this rule is altering pieces that are already in very poor condition, which brings me to my second point. I would ask that you avoid garments that are in good condition; many times, garments with many rips, tears, or other faults can be purchased very inexpensively at antique stores and markets. Once repaired and donned, no one will be able to tell they once were in poor shape.

Even while wearing poor condition pieces, however, it is wise to avoid sitting in beaded dresses, dancing in fragile silk, or walking in delicate silk or satin shoes. Its also an excellent idea to wear protective undergarments; a full slip (with sleeves and dress shields, unless you're wearing a sleeveless dress) is of great help in protecting vintage garments from perspiration and other body chemicals.

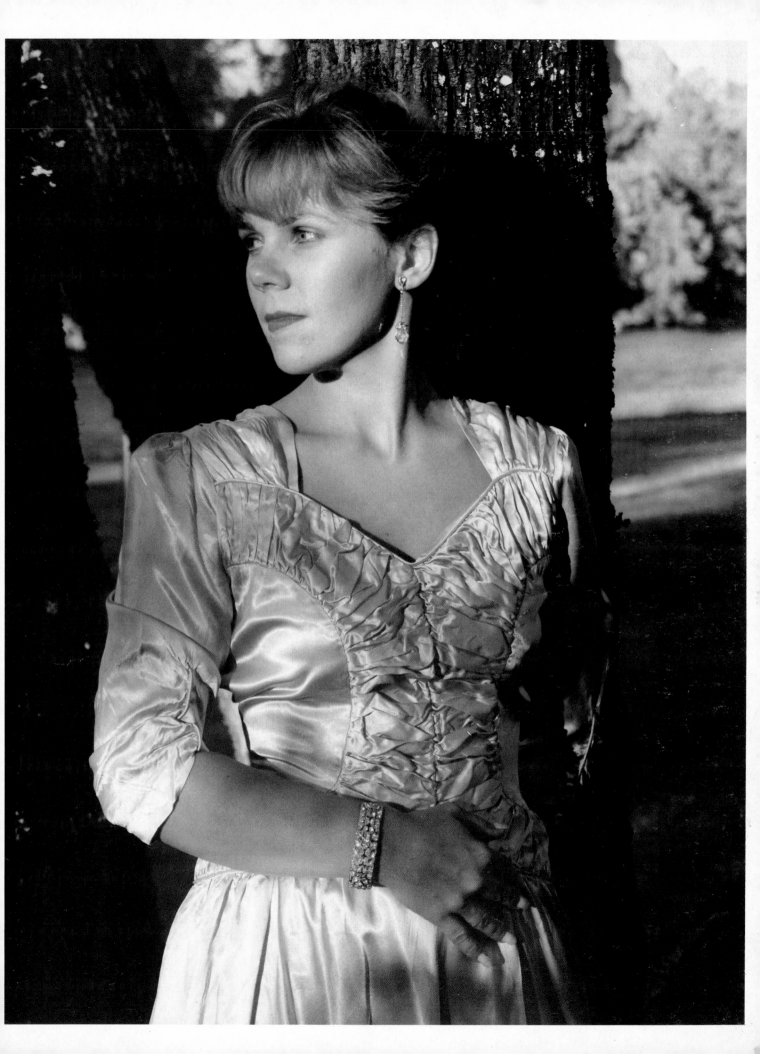

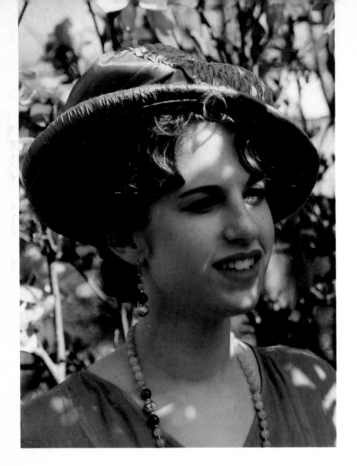

In the 1920s hats were a coveted fashion accessory.

FAKES

Like every other type of collectible, fakes can be found at shops and sales marked and priced as originals. Novice collectors may have difficulty discerning such fakes from originals, but since most vintage fashion "fakes" are actually theatrical costumes, some clues as to authenticity may be found. Most notably, modern notions (such as nylon zippers) are clues that the garment is not authentic. But clouding this area is the fact that authentic garments are sometimes used by theaters with the addition of modern zippers, a dash of modern lace, and a little speedy alteration. Sometimes these garments can be restored and make important additions to a collection—but it takes an eye that is thoroughly familiar with the real thing to spot the difference between a "fake" and a masquerading original.

The best advice for beginning collectors is to trust your instincts. Study the photographs in this book carefully, and visit vintage clothing shops to get familiar with authentic garments. Then, when shopping, use a careful eye and your best judgment. If something tells you that the fabric of a certain dress just seems too modern to be from 1920, then walk away.

BUYING KNOW-HOW

Beginning collectors will almost certainly buy a few "mistakes." However, keeping an eye out for condition is one of the best ways collectors can protect themselves. While a few small holes or rips in a garment might be acceptable, large rips or holes (or a large *number* of rips and holes) are definitely to be avoided. To be sure you aren't buying a garment that will fall to pieces once you get it home (believe me, it has happened!), hold it up to the light. If you can detect any tiny "pin holes" in the fabric, that garment is on the verge of deteriorating.

Collectors should also avoid garments that have been altered. Though some garments will have what curators refer to as "acceptable" repairs made by the original wearers, alterations like iron-on tape patching a moth-hole or nylon zippers inserted into plackets are clearly the work of modern hands and therefore make the garment less valuable.

Furs—though generally difficult to find because of current social attitudes—are also questionable investments. It is extremely difficult for private collectors to preserve fur well, and often vintage furs are already brittle and dry. Ultimately, private collectors can expect most garments made entirely of (or even mostly of) fur to last only about forty years. If you decide to add furs to your collection, do so only because you love the garments, and understand that they probably won't last like the rest of your collection.

FABRICS & REALITY

Wouldn't it be wonderful if collectors could learn the properties of all fabrics so that they could be identified and treated properly once in a collection? Unfortunately, in order to identify most vintage fabrics with much certainty, collectors either need to conduct burn tests or microscopic analysis. Neither is very practical. Fiber content labels were not, as a rule, sewn into clothing until mandated by law in the 1940s; even when content labels *are* found in vintage clothes, fabric types are often obscured because each manufacturer had its own name for fabric types. (For instance, "Koda" was the name for a rayon/acetate blend from one manufacturer, while another manufacturer called the same blend "Sacony-Ciella".)

Collectors do eventually develop a feel for fabrics. After several years of collecting, you will be able to spot cottons, silks, and rayons—but there will always be unidentifiable fabrics. This is particularly true in the 1920s, 1930s, and 1940s, when many man-made fibers were created.

SILK: A SPECIAL CONCERN

While many glorious fashions were created in smooth, supple silk, this fabric is an iffy investment for collectors. In your hunt for vintage clothing, you will no doubt run across garments that appear shredded or rotted away. Experts refer to this as "shattering"—and no matter how well cared for, all silks that were finished or "weighed" with certain chemical properties will eventually destroy themselves in this manner.

If you buy vintage silk garments, realize that their value may decrease with age. Then, since it is virtually impossible for collectors to tell the difference between a silk that will shatter and one that may not, its wise to treat every silk garment as if it *will*. The shattering process is best slowed down by not allowing the silk to touch itself—which means padding the garment with white unbleached muslin. If the garment is particularly fragile and lined in a fabric other than silk, turn the garment inside out while in storage, and carefully stuff it with muslin. With meticulous care, many vintage silk garments can last as long as non-silk garments.

STORAGE

If cared for properly, vintage clothing will not only increase in value, but will last for future generations to enjoy and learn from. One of the most important things you can do to protect your collection is to find a proper home for it. Unlike modern, everyday clothes, vintage fashions should rarely be hung. Occasionally, if space is limited and a dress or blouse is very light-weight, placing it on a well-padded hanger is permissible. All other garments, however, should be stored flat. Absolutely *never* hang bias-cut or beaded garments. The first will stretch out of shape; the latter are so heavy they will eventually tear at the shoulder and neck areas.

Find a trunk, a dresser, or some boxes that are large enough to hold several garments. Line them with unbleached muslin or a clean white sheet, then layer the garments (heaviest on bottom) inside the boxes. Separate the garments from each other with several layers of acid-free tissue from an art supply store (this type of tissue won't cause yellow spots to appear on vintage clothing the way regular tissue paper will). Pad any necessary folds in the garment with crumpled-up acid-free tissue paper to prevent permanent fold lines and wrinkles from appearing. Shoes, hats, and purses should also be gently stuffed with acid-free tissue, then wrapped in unbleached muslin.

You will need to replace your acid-free tissue about once a year. It is also an excellent idea to refold stored garments

A soft evening suit from the early 1940s. *Courtesy of The Very Little Theatre.*

13

every six months or so, as further protection against permanent fold lines. Because fabrics need to breathe in order to remain healthy, *never* place any vintage garment in a plastic bag. If you feel your collection needs extra protection from dust or dirt, use a white cotton garment bag.

CLEANING

When you acquire any piece of vintage clothing, ask the previous owner whether or not the garment was recently cleaned. If their answer is yes, do not clean the garment again; cleaning is very hard on old fabrics, which are always more fragile than they appear. In fact, unless the garment is noticeably dirty, cleaning should be avoided altogether.

Many times, a vintage garment that isn't actually dirty may smell musty. This can be remedied by airing the garment either on a bed or table in a room where all the windows have been opened, or (less preferably) outside on a white cotton sheet. In either case, the garment should be kept away from direct sunlight, which is a great destroyer of old fabrics. If any musty odors persist, steam the garment with a hand-held fabric steamer (available at most drugstores) while it hangs on a well-padded hanger. Be prepared for the pungent odor. After thoroughly steaming the garment, remove it from the hanger and air it again.

Washing vintage garments can be risky, since many synthetic fabrics were used from the 1920s forward. Unlike all-natural cottons, many man-made fabrics from this period will shrivel up if washed. If you are uncertain if it is safe to wash any garment, first test it for color-fastness. Dip a white washcloth into luke-warm water and the soap you intend to use. (This, by the way, should not be regular detergent or soap. Even products marketed as "gentle" are much too harsh for vintage textiles. Instead, use either Orvus—most easily found in fabric and sewing shops under the brand name "Quilt Care"—or a little Neutrogena liquid face soap.) Next, *lightly* rub the washcloth onto a hidden inner seam allowance. If any color appears on the washcloth, the garment is not color-fast and cannot be washed. Allow the tested area to dry thoroughly, then examine it carefully for any shriveling.

If the garment is color-fast and does not shrivel in your test, it is probably safe to wash it. But don't just toss the garment into the washing machine; much gentler care is needed. First, place a pillowcase at the bottom of a sink (or a large white sheet at the bottom of a bathtub), and fill it slowly with lukewarm water, adding only enough soap to give gentle bubbles; too many bubbles will only make your job more difficult. Now gently lower

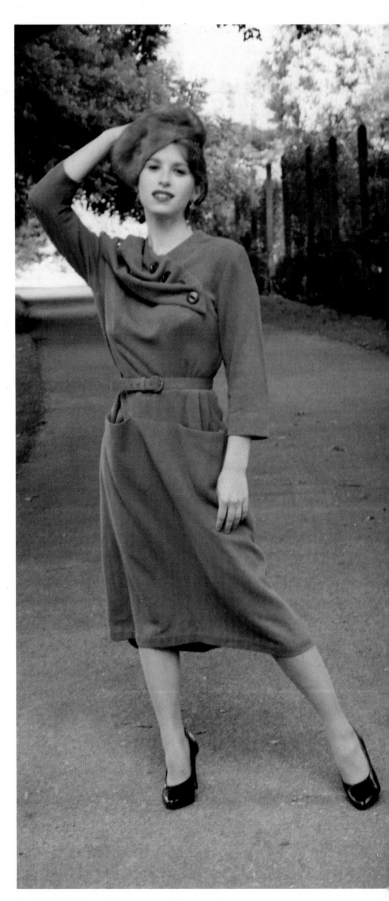

What today would be referred to as "classic" styles emerged in the 1940s. *Courtesy of The Very Little Theatre.*

14

the garment into the water and agitate by hand. Do not allow the garment to sit in the water for more than a half hour, since any dirt that has fallen off the garment will tend to seep back into the fabric after thirty minutes. Remove the garment from the water by lifting up two edges of the pillowcase or sheet. Drain the sink or tub. To rinse the garment, lower the pillowcase or sheet back into the basin and fill it slowly with lukewarm water. Gently press the bubbles out of the garment—do not squeeze or twist. Repeat this process until all the bubbles have been removed.

To dry a hand-washed garment, place it on a clean screen (either the kind created for drying sweaters or, for larger items, a piece of fiberglass screening purchased at a hardware store). Be certain any rough edges on the screening are covered thoroughly with masking tape, and keep the garment out of direct sunlight.

Woolens, sweaters, beaded items, acetates, rayons, most silks, and garments with metal zippers should never be washed. If necessary, most vintage clothes can be dry-cleaned—but be certain to choose a cleaner who either specializes in delicate bridal wear or is recommended by a local museum. Ask the cleaner to place the garment in a mesh bag before running it through his machines—or, create your own "bag" by sandwiching the garment between two layers of unbleached muslin and basting the layers together (creating an outline of the garment). Finally, ask the cleaner to run your garment through his machinery only *after* he has changed to fresh solvent.

Still, while dry-cleaning may seem to be the easy answer to cleaning vintage fashions, it can be just as risky as other washing methods. In many instances, the chemicals used in the dry-cleaning process make old fabrics more brittle and more likely to rip and tear. Silks in particular seem to be more prone to shattering (and some vintage fabrics will completely disintegrate) after being dry-cleaned.

Once your vintage fashions are cleaned, if they seem wrinkled and in need of pressing, use a hand-held fabric steamer. If you *must* iron any garment, use only a steam iron on a low setting, along with a good press cloth—otherwise many vintage fabrics will take on shine.

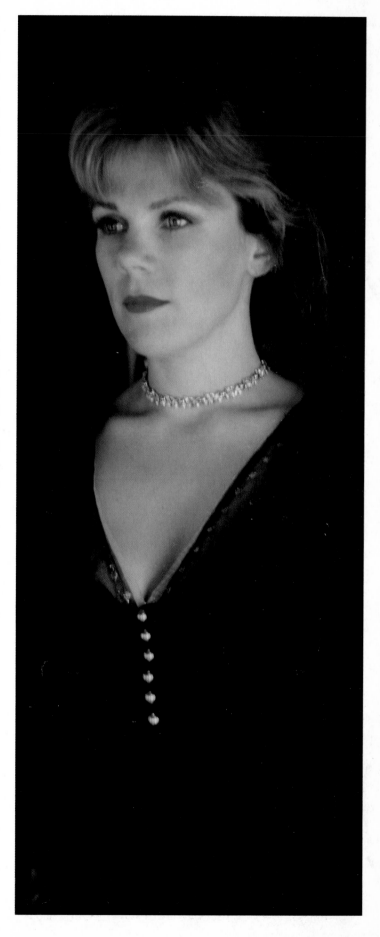

In the 1930s, subtle, elegant fashions prevailed in evening wear.

DOCUMENTATION & VALUE

A collection that is documented tends to be perceived as more valuable by others—including those who may eventually acquire it or a piece of it. A well-documented collection is also easier to appraise and will please your insurance agent. And documentation can *increase* the actual value of your collection—sometimes as much as ten percent. Perhaps most importantly, documentation will help you to focus on what direction your collection is heading in and what you may wish to focus on in the future.

If you already have a large collection, taking the first few steps toward documentation may seem daunting—but it isn't as awful as it may at first seem. And once your exsisting collection is documented, it won't take much time at all to document newcomers. If you are just beginning to collect, documentation has the further advantage of teaching you "hands on" a great deal about vintage fashions.

CREATING YOUR "BRAG BOOK"

The first step toward good documentation is labeling and coding. This is easily done by cutting strips of unbleached muslin or twill tape, then marking them with a code number in permanent ink and tacking them into the garment.

Over the years, museums have developed a simple, yet effective method of giving separate codes for each garment, which private collectors can easily adopt; if I, for instance, had a 1930s chiffon dress that I had purchased in November of 1995, I would code that garment: 95:11 (that is, the year 1995, the month of November). If you are a heavy–duty purchaser, you may also wish to add the *day* to your code. For example: 95.11.25 (1995, the month of November, the 25th day). Another important aspect of coding is adding some indication of where you purchased the garment. For example, the addition of the initials PVC to the end of any code in my collection indicates that I purchased the item from a local dealer called Persona Vintage Clothing. Keep a list of these initials (and the names, addresses, and phone numbers of the dealers). Finally, add an acquisition number to your code. If, for example, that 1930s chiffon dress was the ninetieth garment I had purchased for my collection, its code would be 95.11.25.PVC.90.

While labeling your collection, its also a good idea to make a rough sketch of where every item in your collection lays within your storage area. This will prevent needless rummaging when you're looking for a specific piece.

Now you can get down to actually creating your documentation book (what I affectionately refer to as a "brag book"). This can be as simple or elaborate as you like. Probably the most functional brag book consists of a three–ring binder with 8.5 by 11 inch paper inserted into plastic protective sheets. Type (or neatly handwrite) all pertinent information about the item onto your sheet, including: A description of the garment, its era, how much you paid for it, its history (who wore it and when, if you can find out), its condition, and how it was restored and cleaned. Add a photograph of the garment, plus photocopies from any relevant magazines or books.

Be sure to include the sketch of your storage area in your brag book, in addition to your dealer coding and addresses. This is also an ideal place to keep your insurance information, appraisals, bills of sale, or any other papers pertinent to your collection.

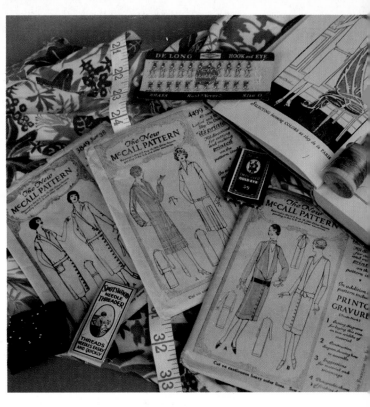

Sewing patterns and other similar items are useful to vintage clothing collectors. Shown here are three McCall patterns from the first half of the twenties, a sewing reference book published by Butterick Pattern Company in 1927, and various sewing notions, including hook and eye sets and needles in their original packaging.

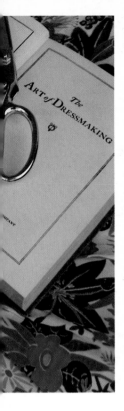

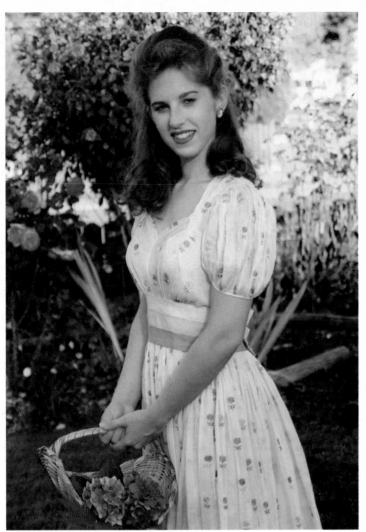

Garment: Day Dress   Acquisition #: 90.2.OF.90

Era/Date: circa 1947
Description: Day dress with sweetheart neckline, full, long skirt,
     three-ribbon waistband, and embroidered flowers.
Color: White with vari-colored ribbons and flowers.
Fabrics: Fine cotton lawn.

Source: Old Friends Vintage Clothing (Eugene, Oregon), $45

Condition: Excellent.

Treatments: Was dry-cleaned by dealer.

Restoration: None.

Size: 6 (small through the shoulders)

Comments:

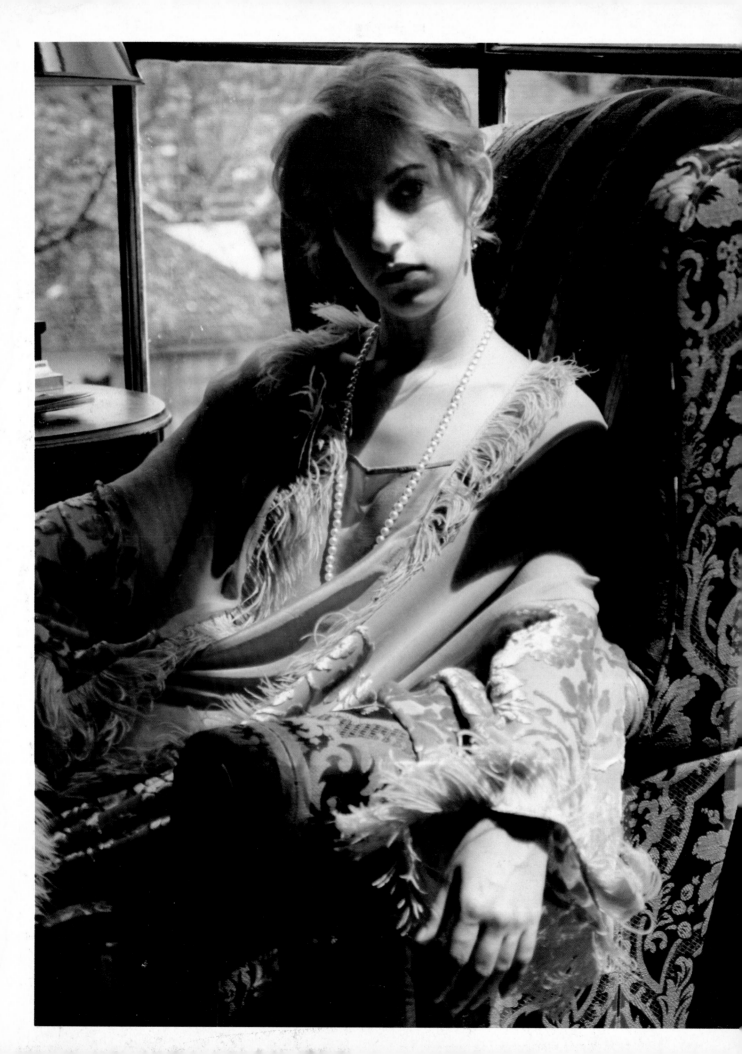

The wedding gown was one of the few articles of women's clothing not subject to rationing restrictions during World War II. *Courtesy of Dorothy Wright.*

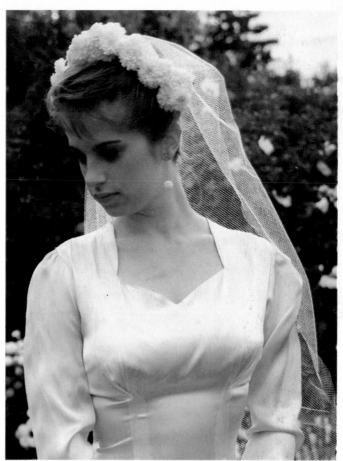

A day suit from the early 1940s. Simple and clean-cut, it is typical of the period. *Courtesy of The Very Little Theatre.*

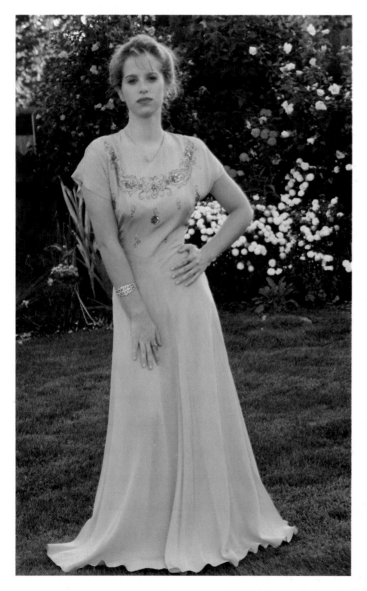

By evening, simple dresses embellished with beading were *the* thing to wear in the forties. *Courtesy of The Very Little Theatre.*

Previous Page:

Whether trimmed with beads, lace, embroidery, or marabou feathers, the fashions of the 1920s through 1940s are some of the most readily available fashion collectibles around. *Courtesy of Persona Vintage Clothing.*

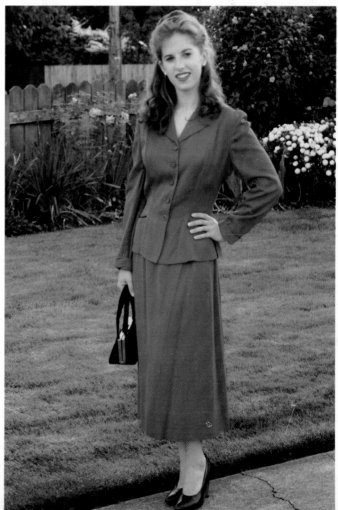

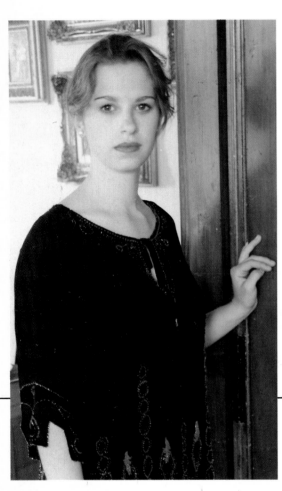

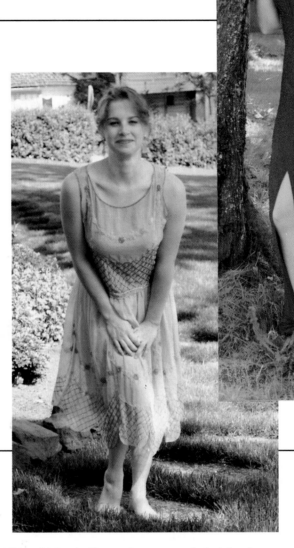

Beading was a particularly popular trimming in the 1920s. *Courtesy of The Very Little Theatre.*

Elaborately beaded flapper dresses are a collector's favorite. *Courtesy of The Very Little Theatre.*

In the forties, wearing sophisticated dancing dresses was an important part of "welcoming" soldiers on furlough. *Courtesy of The Very Little Theatre.*

Boudoir caps from the 1920s are both exquisitely detailed and highly collectible. *Courtesy of The Very Little Theatre.*

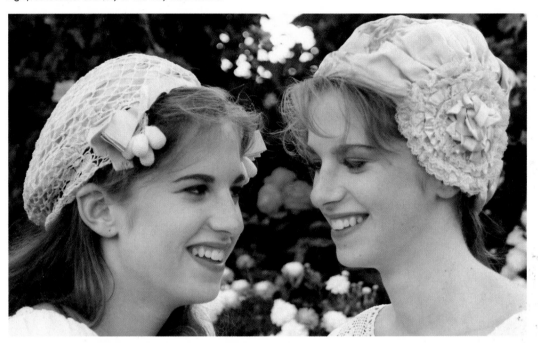

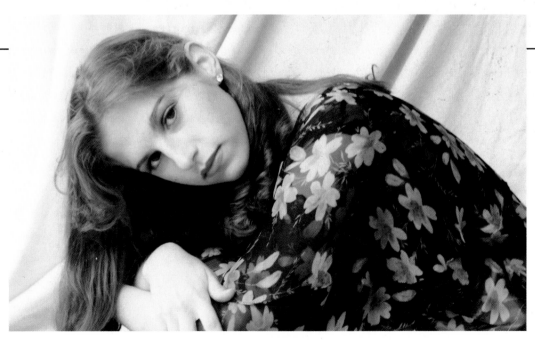

Soft and sheer dresses from the 1930s are also much sought after by vintage fashion collectors. *Courtesy of The Very Little Theatre.*

CHAPTER TWO

IDENTIFICATION & DATING

Though some collectors are blissfully content to acquire fashions that merely please them—with no thought about identifying the pieces in any way—most collectors will find that in order to make certain they know exactly what they are buying, they must know at least a little about identification. (Who wants to buy a fringed 1960s dress, thinking it's a 1920s flapper dress?)

This book guides you step by step through the twenties, thirties, and forties, helping you to identify and date your collection through descriptions and illustrations of both the *exterior* and *interior* of vintage garments. Though this book contains photographs from period fashion magazines and other similar sources, this should not keep you from amassing your own collection of them. Fashion plates can be especially useful (though some plates from the twenties forward tend to be less useful than fashion plates from earlier eras, because they are distorted and "arty"). Fashion magazines (such as *Vogue* and *Harper's Bazaar* for ultra-fashionable styles, or *Glamour, Mademoiselle,* and *Ladies' Home Journal* for more down-to-earth fashions), sewing patterns (from any of the hundreds of companies that produced them, including Butterick, Hollywood, and Vogue), mail-order fashion catalogs (such as Sears), pattern catalogs (like *Pictorial Review Patterns*), and period photographs are all collectible in their own right and will help you to better understand and identify the actual fashions you collect.

It's In The Details

When attempting to date any garment, study it for details like those described in each chapter of this book. Examining the *inside* of the garment is just as important as examining the outside, so don't skip over information about construction and craftsmanship. Remember too that you'll probably never find an *exact* picture or description of any garment in your collec-

tion; most vintage garments in existence today are one of a kind (even if they may have been mass-produced in the past). Instead, look for strong similarities in necklines, waistlines, sleeve styles, etcetera.

Other Clues

Identification can begin the moment you acquire a piece. Always ask the previous owner of the garment whether they know anything about the garment's past; you might be surprised how many people (including dealers) have family stories that accompany garments. Though oral histories aren't always accurate, they are nonetheless interesting and often enlightening. If you can document those stories with photographs of the original owner (preferably wearing the garment), newspaper clippings, etcetera, it will also add value to the garment itself.

Some other clues—which may not at first be obvious—can be detected directly from the garment itself. Buttons and hooks and eyes, for example, should always be examined carefully with a magnifying glass. Sometimes actual dates are embossed on such fastenings; occasionally, manufacture names are also imprinted on them.

Zippers, more than any other type of fastening, are particularly telling. Though the zipper was patented in the late nineteenth century and was used in some sportsclothes in the 'teens, it wasn't until 1929–1930 that it began to appear in women's clothes. Even then, however, only a few élan designers, such as Schiaparelli, used the new contraption. In reality, it wasn't until late in the 1930s that the zipper was in fairly regular use in women's dress.

If you find a garment that has a zipper, and if indeed the garment dates to the thirties or forties, it will have a rather heavy, clunky metal zipper, which will almost certainly be on the side of the garment (*not* running straight down the back). Though it is possible a nylon or polyester zipper was used to replace an original metal zipper, most often such modern fastenings are a definite clue that the garment dates to a later period.

Previous page:
Refined wedding gowns were typical in the 1940s. *Courtesy of Marianine's Vintage Chic.*

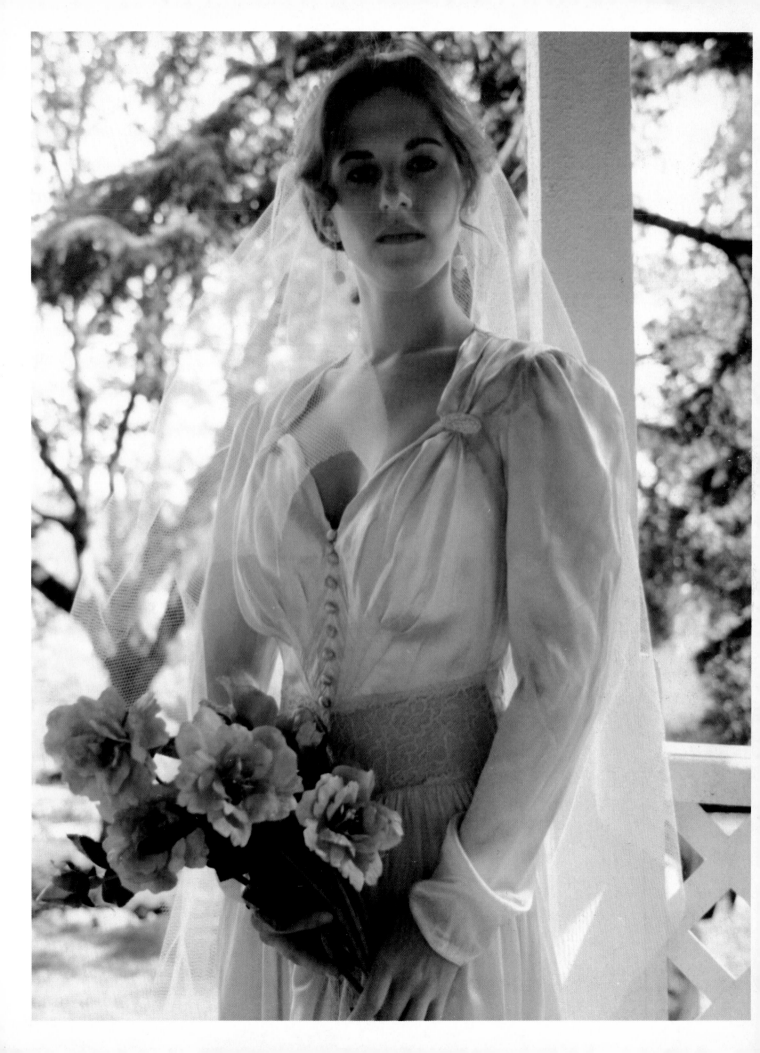

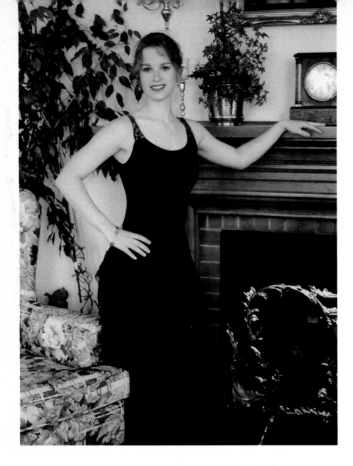

Though this gown has many characteristics of a 1920s dress, the smooth fit, flounces, and long length date it to the early 1930s. *Courtesy of Persona Vintage Clothing.*

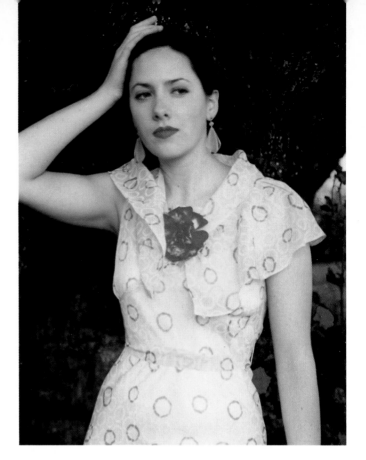

Ethnic looks—including those in a Latin vein—prevailed through most of the 1920s through 1940s. *Courtesy of Persona Vintage Clothing.*

Some fabrics, too, are telling. For example, rayon that dates from before 1950 feels more silky, thin, and drapable than rayon from after 1950. Fabrics woven with metals were also occasionally used in vintage clothing—especially those from the 1920s. These metals had a tendency to tarnish, while modern metallics are coated in transparent plastic in order to prevent tarnishing. Therefore, a metallic fabric that has no tarnishing whatsoever is almost certainly modern.

LABELS

Though labels rarely appear in pre–1920 garments (unless the garment is the creation of a couture designer), labels are a factor in fashions from the twenties forward. Not all garments from the era have labels (perhaps they were removed because they annoyed the original wearer, or, more likely, the garments were home–made or sewn by a local seamstress), but labels from mass–producers and department stores like Jordan Marsh or Macy's are interesting and are sometimes helpful in dating garments. References on labels to "NRA" (the National Recovery Administration) date to the Depression, and notations such as "Manufactured Under Fair Labor Standards" date to the forties.

On the other hand, collectors should take couture designer labels with a grain of salt. In the 1920s–1940s period, it was notoriously known that labels were removed from couture garments and sewn into non-couture clothes. Department stores also used to remove designer labels and replace them with their own (which was legal in those days). Therefore, a vintage garment with a Chanel label may not actually be an authentic Chanel garment, and a vintage garment without a couture designer label may (I repeat, *may*) actually be a couture garment.

If you are intent on identifying couture garments, look for quality rather than labels. Garments that are largely hand-sewn, have hand-overcast seams, covered snaps, hand-finished facings, or bound or hand-worked buttonholes are almost certainly couture. By the 1920s almost all garments *except* those made by couture designers were machine-sewn. Still, even couture clothes may have a few machine-stitched seams, so check several areas of the garment. In order to distinguish between machine- and hand-sewing, study several seams under a magnifying glass. If adjoining stitches seem to come out of the same hole, the seam was machine-stitched—*unless* the stitches on the underside overlap, in which case the seam was hand-stitched with a technique called backstitching.

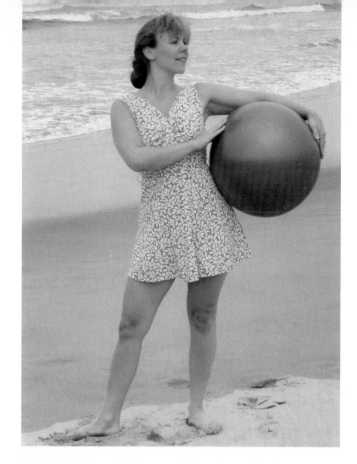

In the 1940s, bathing suits often resembled sundresses. *Courtesy of The Very Little Theatre.*

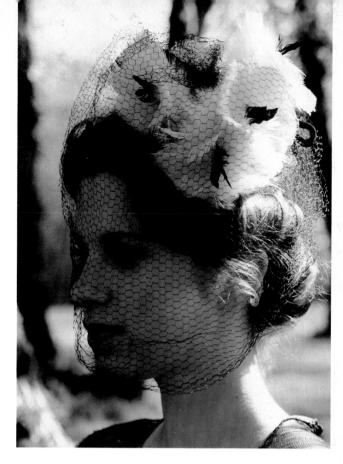

Throughout the twenties, thirties, and forties, hat styles varied enormously. *Courtesy of The Very Little Theatre.*

Even so, vintage couture designs—if you can afford them—can be dubious investments. Fads drastically raise and lower selling prices on couture garments; one year Dior and Patou garments will be popular and sell for extremely high prices, while another year Vionnet and Schiaparelli are favored, and Dior and Patou designs drop in value. Such roller coaster pricing very rarely occurs with "non-designer" fashions.

The sleek, long-line look of this dress may be reminiscent of the 1930s, but the defined waistline and beaded bodice date it to the early 1940s. *Courtesy of The Very Little Theatre.*

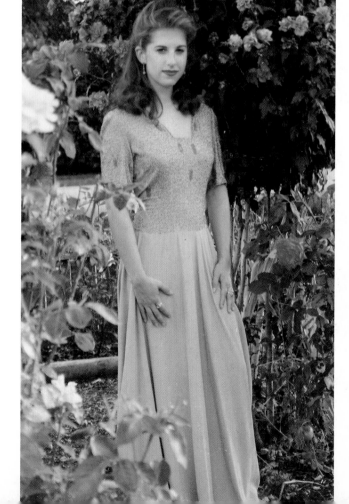

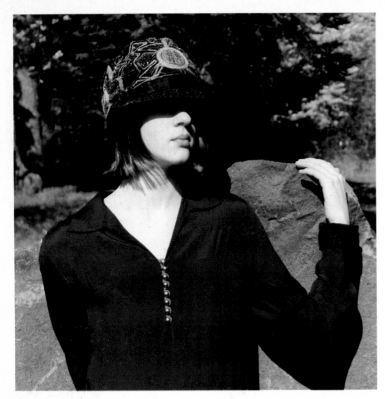

Undeniably flapper in era and in style. *Courtesy of The Very Little Theatre.*

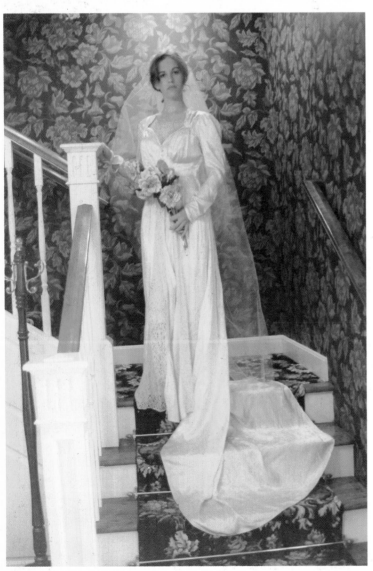

Subtle details like the drape of the wedding gown's sweetheart neckline and the attached dress clips of tiny faux pearls add up to elegance. *Courtesy of Marianine's Vintage Chic.*

Refined wedding gowns with long, full trains were typical in the 1940s. *Courtesy of Marianine's Vintage Chic.*

Following Page:

In the thirties and forties, neo-Victorian styles appeared in small doses. This rich taffeta dress combines Victorian femininity with Latin flamenco style. *Courtesy of The Very Little Theatre.*

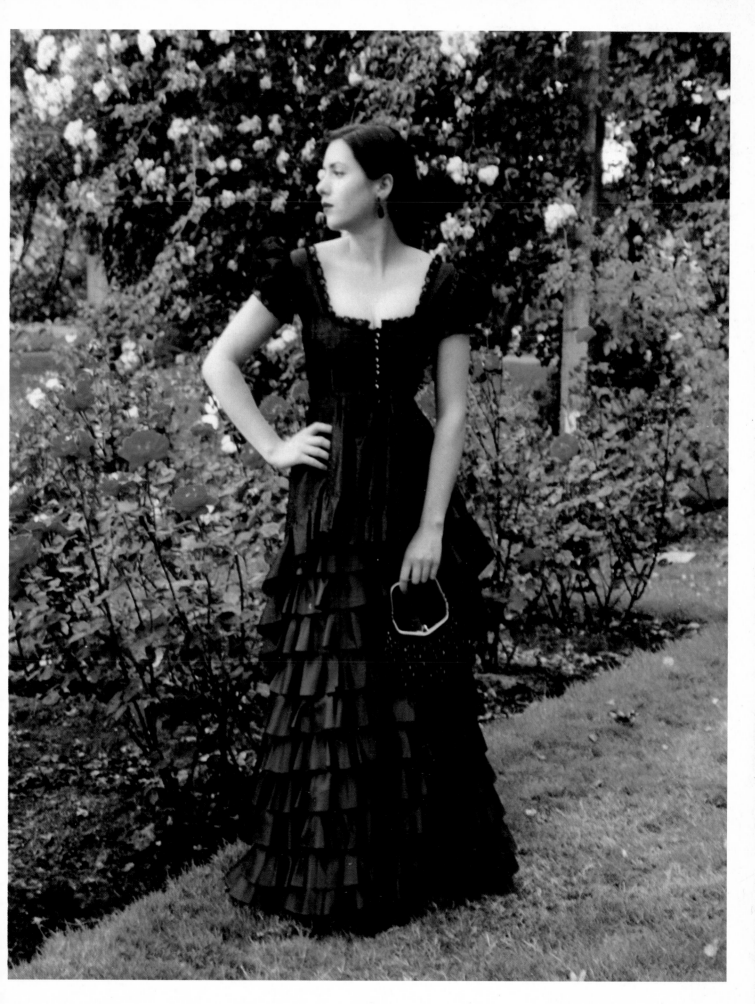

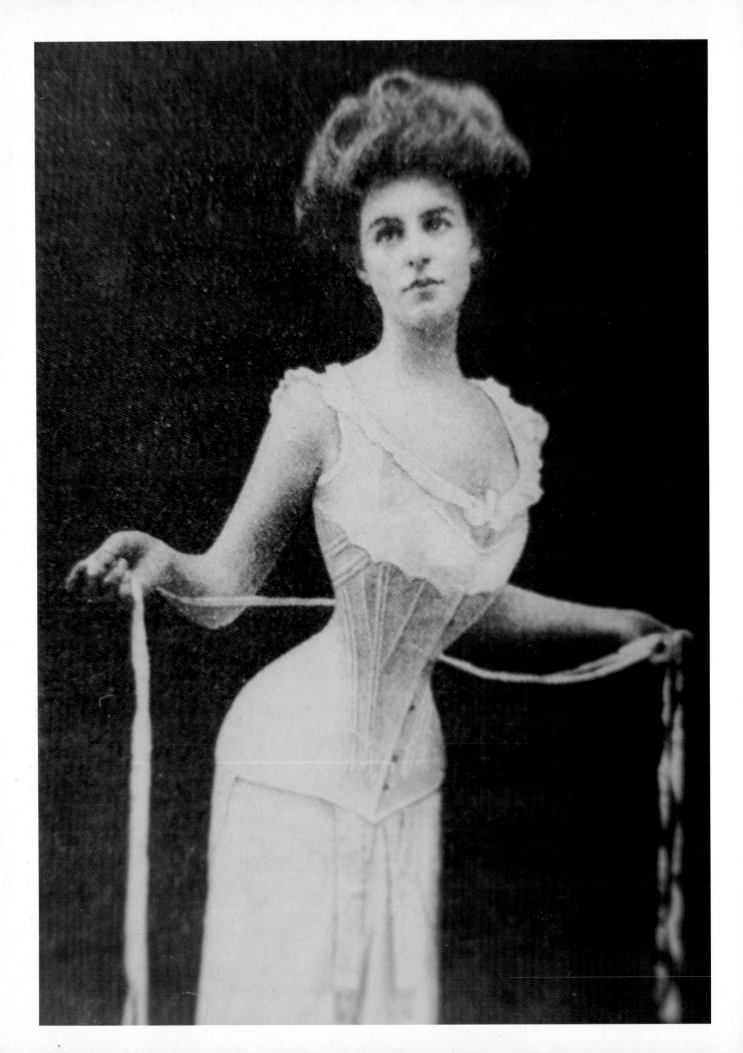

CHAPTER 3

THE BREAKING DAM

*"All things must change
To something new, to something strange"*
—Longfellow

Starting in the mid-Victorian era, the dress reform movement crept along with only minor success. Most everyone seemed to agree some sort of change towards practicality and comfort was necessary in women's clothing, but no one was able to find an acceptable solution; women refused to sacrifice fashion and beauty for the sake of comfort. Yet, as the 'teens pressed forward, a sudden, revolutionary change in women's dress took hold. No one person or group had advocated or pushed this change—so why *did* the change occur? The answer is helpful in understanding the trends of the 1920s through 1940s.

At the turn of the century, when the women's rights movement was at its zenith, women shed their bell-shaped, wasp-waisted, oddly humped attire. Still, rows of tiny hooks and eyes trailed down their backs, skirts consisting of enormous amounts of fabric swathed their legs, and one of the most confining corsets in history shaped their body into a queer S–curve.

When the Great War disrupted traditional life, many men left the workforce for the battlefield, and women found unsurpassed opportunity in the business world. Though their corsets were still long and boned, women shed most of their petticoats and adopted the largely angular, severe clothing so typical of the 'teens. Suits were staples, skirts were usually slender, box–like, and often "hobbling" (some fashionable women even wore "shackles" around their ankles, in order to ensure they took dainty steps). Evening styles were draped, emphasizing a long, lean line, and were more sophisticated than had been seen in centuries. Still, while the new fashions *appeared* mostly modern and emancipating, they were actually uncomfortable and confining: boned, tightly lined, and difficult to walk in.

Previous Page:

In the early 1900s, women encased themselves in what was one of the most confining corsets ever worn: long, rigid, and S-shaped.

When the war ended, women were not willing to give up what little freedom they had acquired. Though urged to leave the businesses they had sustained during war years, many women refused—causing much angst in the male populous. One particular man—named, appropriately, General Alarm—fought outspokenly to have women removed from business. Not only were women stealing the best jobs, the popular war hero claimed, but they had the nerve to adopt men's vices, too, including swearing and smoking. Feeling that men's sacred territory was being invaded, he even chastised women for adopting "every article of [man's] attire, down to, and including, his sox!" A good number of women held fast to their careers, however, and were still fighting for (and soon won) their suffrage. As new ideas about women began emerging, it was only natural women's clothes should change, too.

As early as 1914, an eccentric named Nina Wilcox Putnam (still in her early twenties) had been told she was dying of T.B. Instead of taking to her sickbed as prescribed, she moved to the roof of her New York City apartment building and lived in a tent. This, Putnam claimed, saved her life and gave her time to invent a new style: the tubular dress. This new style—the predecessor to the slip of a dress worn in the twenties—was made simply by folding a length of cloth in half, cutting a hole for the head, then sewing up the sides, leaving holes for arms. Putnam then lightly tucked in the waist with a belt. The entire process took her only a half hour and cost her a mere $2 (as compared to $10 for the average ready-made dress). But women, still clinging to Victorian ideals, were not eager to accept her new dress style. Then why did they embrace it in 1920?

As one contemporary writer, Mark Sullivan, observed: "Changes in social standards have [usually] been slow, gradual, almost imperceptible until long afterwards. In America, during the 1920s, the old codes went out like the breaking of a dam. More correctly, what happened was an explosion." Then—as

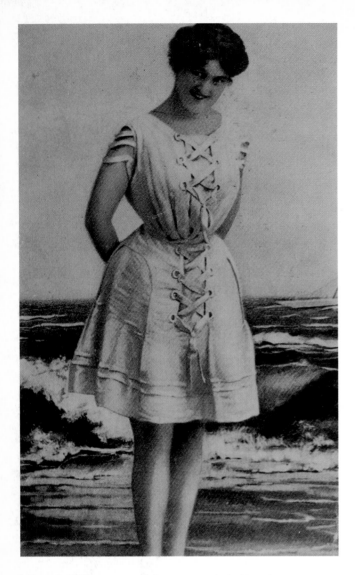

In the early 1900s, corsets were worn even under bathing suits. The idea was to achieve the "bathing beauty" look—not necessarily to be practical.

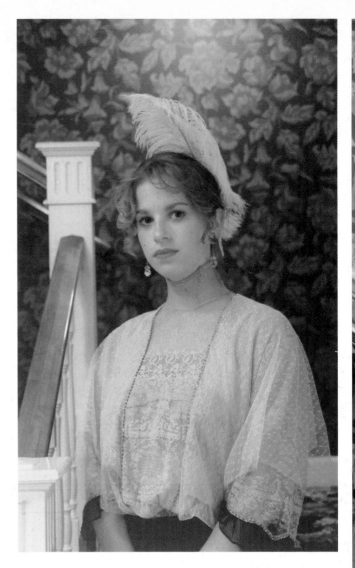

now—there was much speculation as to why this "dam" burst open: was it feminism, modernism, too much wealth, or new central heating that made women adopt short–short skirts and sleeveless dresses? More probably, it was youthful disillusionment—the likes of which wouldn't be seen again until the 1960s. As Mr. Sullivan put it, Victorian "totems" and social practices were found to be hypocritical:

> "The younger generation looked into those old totems, found them fakes, and with a back slap of the hand knocked them over. The younger generation went, in their belated adolescence, through the moral equivalent of finding out about Santa Claus. They found that the standards and convictions and rules before which publicly we had knelt down, did not conform at all with our private convictions or our personal practices...Thereupon the young people set up some new standards of their own."

1919 was a year of great change. For the first time, dresses designed specifically for maternity wear appeared on the market—announcing that, at long last, women weren't expected to go into confinement during the last stages of their pregnancy. Also during that year, the National Federation of Business and Professional Women was organized, and corsets were banished.

Later in 1919, legs began to appear —and while many men made a huff about the new "indecency" of short skirts, one *Literary Digest* reader censured: "Why should the fact that a girl has legs arouse the wrong kind of impulses in a man? Does he think we travel on wheels?"

As if corsetless figures and bared ankles were not enough, "painted ladies" were becoming the norm. *Vogue* confided in 1919: "I have heard, though I did not, myself, witness this, that during the luncheon, at a well-known restaurant recently, a mutual friend of ours...was seen, not only to powder her nose in full view of everybody, but to redden her lips!"

And so, as Sullivan suggested, the new, tempestuous woman tossed aside her cloak of Victorian propriety and sallied forth, brimming with *IT*, to sip cocktails and make whoopee in nightclubs. For reasons both clear and vague, the modern woman was born.

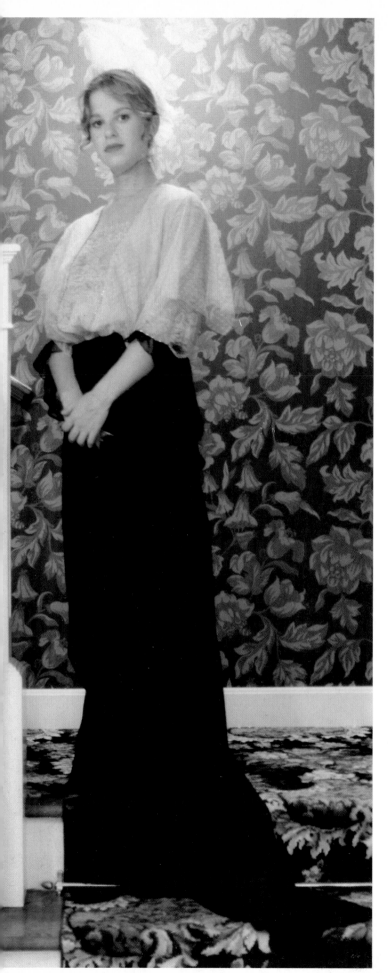

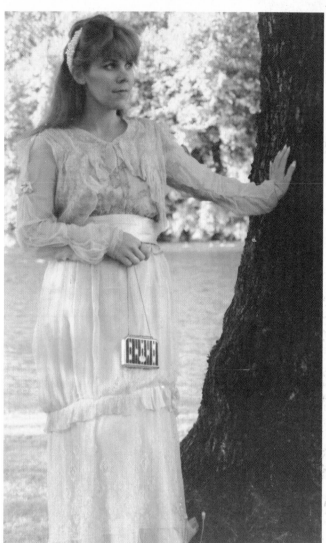

Though 'teens dresses often featured tubular styles, they were far fussier than the minimalist fashions most favored in the 1920s. *Courtesy of The Very Little Theatre.*

Notice the clever use of "illusion" netting; this gave this tubular dress an unprecedented "revealing" look that seems to contradict the high, boned collar and tightly belted waistline. Evening gowns like this one were forerunners of the tubular twenties look. *Courtesy of The Very Little Theatre.*

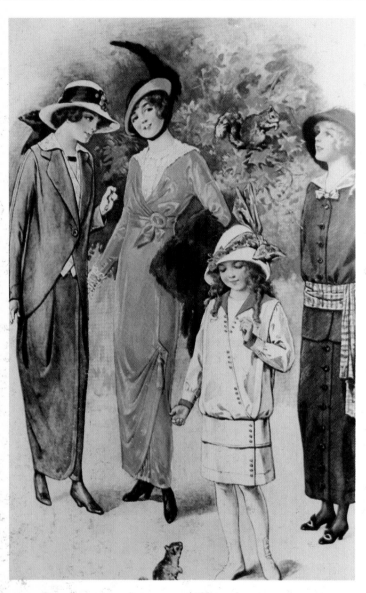

A 'teens fashion plate featuring long, lean styles.

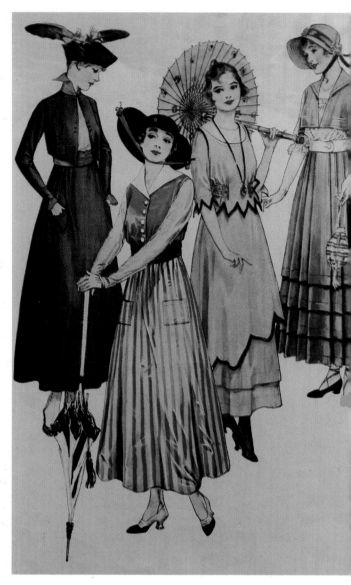

This 'teens fashion plate shows styles that were still very much in the Victorian vein.

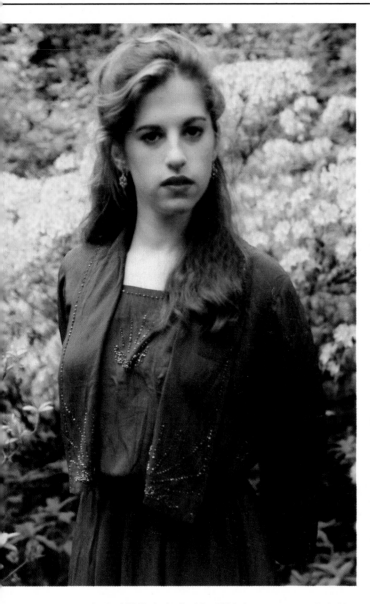

Around 1919, the look of the 1920s began to emerge in fashions like this simple sailor-collar dress. *Courtesy of The Very Little Theatre.*

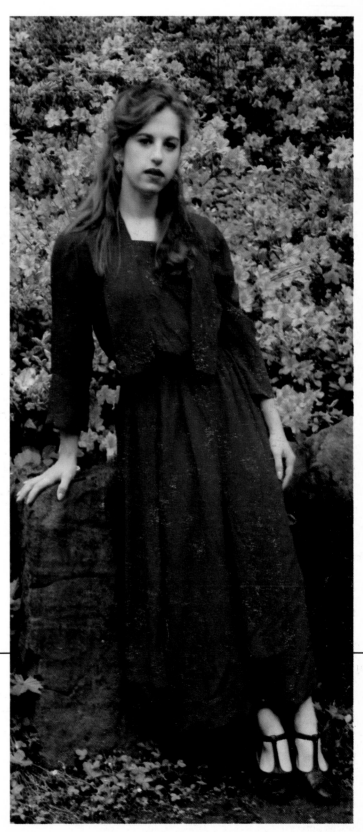

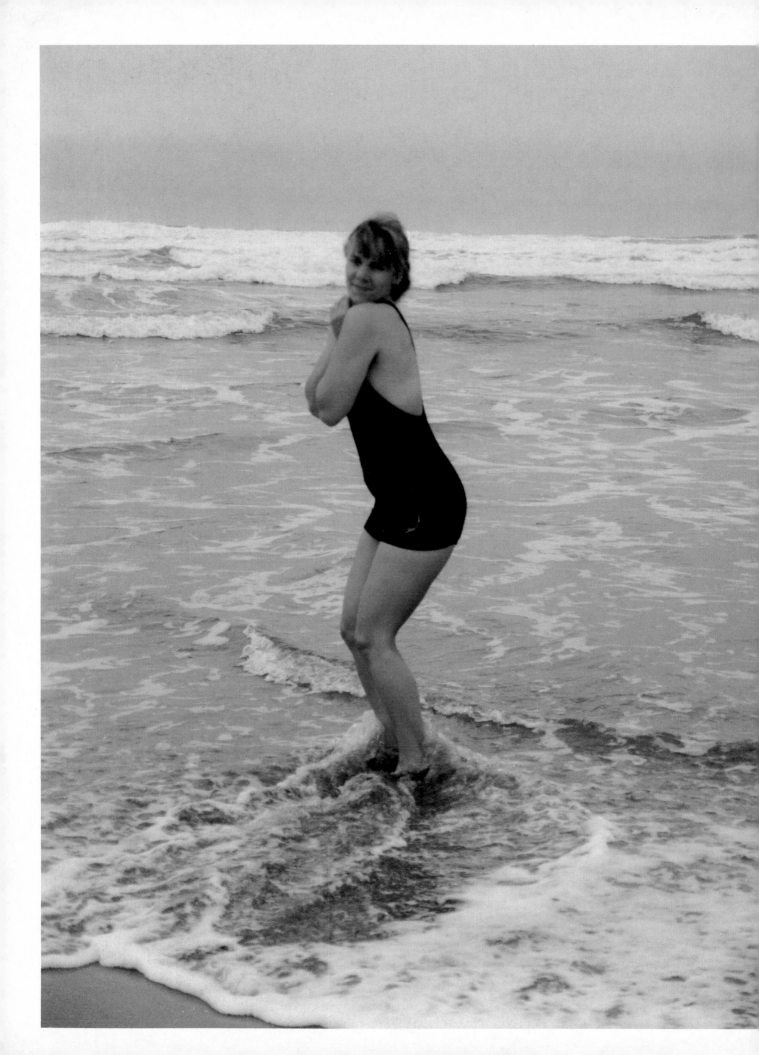

CHAPTER FOUR

1920S: THE TOMBOY

"Off went the corsets, snap went the garters. Roll went the stockings," *The Delineator* wrote in 1928, reflecting on the radical changes in fashion at the beginning of the decade. "Women were free at last. And what funny looking things most of them were! Of course, mummies are funny looking too. Why not? Anybody would be who had been wrapped up and bound down the way women had been for thousands of years."

Indeed, after centuries of corsets and tight, heavy, full clothes, women of the twenties looked like entirely different creatures than they had a mere decade earlier. "Since Eve wandered out of the Garden of Eden attired in a fig leaf, she has seldom gone so slightly clad," one survivor of the Twenties commented. "Dresses were never [before] so short nor cut so low, nor were they ever made of thinner material." As if to place themselves equally with men, women—after centuries of emphasizing their curves—adopted an entirely curveless mode, which later came to be known as the "flapper look." Unfortunately, all but the very thin and ethereal tended to look frumpy in the new, tubular style. Florence Ziegfield, creator of the enormously popular and flamboyant *Ziegfield Follies*, described the new fashionable women thus: "Height—5 ft., Weight—117 pounds, Foot size—5 . . . A girl weighing 100 to 105 pounds has ten more chances of marriage than the 135 pounder, and 25 more chances than the 150—"

In 1925, *New Republic* writer Bruce Bliven described the flapper as nineteen but affecting worldly wisdom. She smoked, drank, got hangovers, and took every opportunity to attend "petting parties." She drove like a lunatic and used vulgarities freely; she wore heavy layers of make-up which gave her a China-doll face of white, punctuated by red cheeks and lips. Her clothes, Bliven stated, "were estimated...by some statistician to weigh two pounds...I doubt they came within half a pound." He went on to say that the flapper "wasn't wearing much this summer...one dress, one step-in, two stockings, two shoes." He ranted further, describing her dress merely as "brief. It is cut low where it might be high, and vice versa. The skirt comes just an inch below her knees, overlapping by a faint

fraction her rolled and twisted stockings...In hot weather [she] reserves the right to discard her stockings."

But despite all the titillating descriptions and social hubbub, the average woman was not nearly so radical. She might use some make-up—yes, she probably bobbed her hair, too. And almost certainly she wore the new–fangled "ready–to–wear" clothes. But the average woman had more modesty than the infamous flapper caricaturized in period cartoons and romanticized by Fitzgerald novels.

DRESSES

In 1920, the average woman still wore fairly wide skirts—though they were a little shorter than those worn in the 'teens. Bustlines were no longer emphasized. Adornment was considered Victorian and therefore vulgar. And by 1921, the tubular, boyish look was definitely beginning to take its hold on fashion. Dresses were often extremely simple in cut—frequently looking more like chemises or slips than dresses. *Vogue* raved over the new style, calling it "practical" and "perfectly adapted to the demands of modern life." Perhaps the magazine's favorite aspect of the new style (and, certainly, they were not alone) was that it was decidedly simple to sew; "the number of these simple frocks that are made in the seclusion of the sewing-room to be worn later with the air of having [been] issued from les Grandes Maisons is," *Vogue* concluded, "one of the secrets of the age."

Chemise dresses could usually be slipped on over the head and could have one or two hooks and eyes or snaps, or absolutely no fastenings. In fact, it can be difficult to tell the front from the back in some twenties chemise dresses. Most often, dresses were cut in one piece—or, occasionally, they consisted of a skirt sewn onto the lowered waistline of a bodice. For those who refused (or simply were not allowed by nature) to go completely flat-chested, bustline darts were still essential; however, such darts ran horizontally from the bust point toward the side seam, rather than in the more traditional vertical line.

Previous page:
A nearly bare-backed bathing suit by Jantzen. Courtesy of The Very Little Theatre.

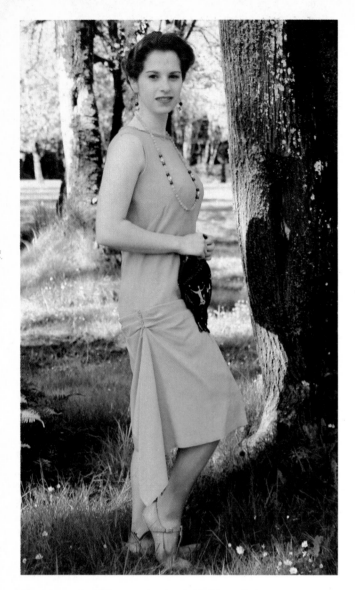

Many dresses had little or no trimming detail. This one features a modest side flounce. *Courtesy of The Very Little Theatre.*

By 1923, the waistline had dropped defiantly to the hip, and could be set off by a wide sash or waistband. By 1924, ensemble dresses, consisting of a carefully matched dress and jacket (or, in some cases, a skirt, blouse, and jacket) were becoming *trés chic*, and enjoyed tremendous popularity all the way through the end of the decade. In 1928, the true tubular look that is so identified with the twenties—without any bands or sashes, falling straight down from the shoulders—was common. By 1929, waistlines made a subtle comeback and the new, more draped and feminine look of the 1930s began to take hold, revealing itself through flounces and frills at the hem.

When the chemise dress became popular, many manufacturers panicked. Desperately, they tried to introduce more traditional styles: long, full skirts, draped dresses, fitted waistlines, and hour-glass curves. "The campaign was on," Mary Allen Hopkins wrote in *New Republic* in 1922. "Flaring, flaunting, flower-beds of skirts, displayed in shop windows, were to tempt the shopper. Lovely wax figures smiled to prove that tight bodices were not uncomfortable." Women were unbelieving, however, and while they flirted with pannier, hooped, and bustle skirt styles (particularly in their evening wear), their allegiance was with the chemise-dress. A dress that was comfortable, easy to care for, and so simple to sew even the most inexperienced seamstress could manage to put it together, was difficult to give up after years of complicated, extravagant styles. Many manufactures (such as those who created heavy skirt bindings) went out of business and many fabric manufactures suffered greatly because they were suddenly unable to sell the enormous quantities of fabric they once did. Trim manufacturers, on the other hand, flourished. To remain interesting, the new, simply-cut dress needed variety in trimming—and variety manufacturers did provide: everything from feathers and pom-pons to spangles, faux pearls, and fur.

Evening dresses, in particular, needed imaginative trimming, and soon beaded evening gowns became the signature of the decade. Such dresses are now a collectors' favorite. Not only are they strikingly "Roaring Twenties," but they are unquestionably pieces of artwork. Before a beaded dress could even be stitched together, panels of fabric (usually airy chiffon or very light weight silk or rayon) were secured into frames, the design marked by hand, and then—by hand and with needle and thread—beaded.

In 1922, the flowing, graceful lines and flowers that had dominated the Art Nouveau age at the turn of the century were squashed by the world's rapture at the opening of King Tutankhamen's tomb. Suddenly, Egyptian-inspired motifs were the rage, whether beaded, stitched with appliqué, or suggested in style lines; hieroglyphics, scarabs, and serpents abounded. With the influence of ancient Egypt came more inspiration from a variety of ethnic groups. Spanish shawls and headdresses, Russian blouses, and Chinese and Japanese kimonos were all the height of sophistication. The Art Deco movement also had a profound affect on fashion, and complimented women's curveless clothes perfectly; geometric prints of all types were considered ultra-modern.

Silk was still the preferred fabric of ladies who could afford it, but rayon—the new man-made wonder billed as "artificial silk"—was heaven-sent for the majority of women. Crepes, georgettes, serges, foulards, voiles, organdies, and chiffons were used frequently by day, while velvets, laces, satins, and chiffons were favored at night. Evening fabrics—in another attempt at "dressing-up" simple, predictable styles—were sometimes also shot with metallic threads.

Skirts

Early in the 1920s, the state of Utah promoted a bill that included fines and imprisonment for women who wore "skirts higher than three inches from the ankle." Utah state was not alone in its shocked concern over the new "short–short" skirt. Indeed, even in the winter, while wrapped up snugly in fashionable furs, the twenties woman allowed her legs to freeze. As if carefully testing the waters, the woman of 1920 began moderately, shortening her skirts only a few inches. By the end of that year, however, her skirts were a never-before-heard-of three to four inches above her ankles—which brought her hemline to mid–calf. By evening, her skirts could be a scandalous seven to eight inches above her ankle.

In 1921, hemlines rushed downwards again, nearly to the ankle (or about six inches from the ankle in some evening wear). From 1922 to 1924, hemlines were worn about two to four inches from the ankle. In 1925, hemlines rushed up again, nearly eight inches from the ankle, and steadily rose until, by 1927, they reached their pinnacle of fifteen inches—just barely below the knee. In 1928, this fell an inch or two, and in 1929, when the stock market crashed, hemlines crashed with it, straight to the floor.

Still, in perfect keeping with the new "freedom" era, skirt lengths were—for the first time in fashion history—arbitrary. "Skirt lengths vary not only according to what designer creates them," *Vogue* stated, "and what lady wears them, but, also, according to the hour of the day when they are worn."

With all this attention thrust onto hemlines, it is something of a wonder that there were any other innovations in skirts of the twenties—but there were. In 1920, some styles of the 'teens still persisted, among them peg–top skirts and A–lines. Still, by 1922, the less full, straighter skirt reigned supreme. In 1923, waistlines dropped resolutely to the hip, remaining there through the rest of the decade. In 1927, while the skirt was at its shortest, the new innovation of an uneven hemline (often longer on the sides than in the front or back, or in the all–over handkerchief style) appeared, and persisted until 1929. Also from 1927 to 1929, pleated skirts—particularly those that were pleated entirely around their circumference—became fashionable.

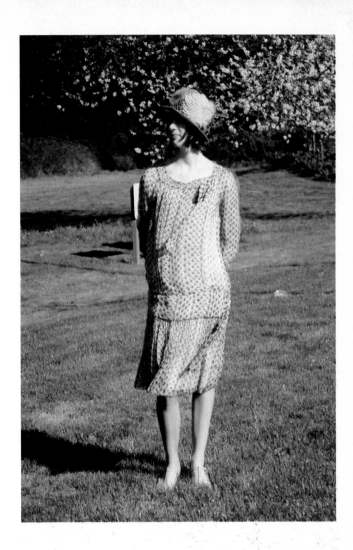

A very common style, featuring an over-blouse and a "skirt" that is actually a chemise-slip with a plain bodice and a print skirt. *Courtesy of The Very Little Theatre.*

Blouses

Blouses with skirts were widely worn for daytime casual wear, especially in the first few years of the twenties. Usually, blouses had wide waistbands and were worn *outside* of the skirt, creating a blouson affect. In the first few years of the decade, this put the bottom of the blouse just barely below the natural waistline; the waistband or tie that loosely belted the blouse followed the same style-lines of fashionable dresses, lowering to the hip around 1921, and falling slightly below the hipline after 1925.

Most blouses had scooping necklines without collars, though jabot-style center panels were favored at mid-decade, and ties were sometimes worn by those enamored of the *garçonne*, man-tailored look. Sailor collars, often worn in the 'teens, continued to be popular, but the latest news in blouses was the Peter Pan collar. Nothing could have been more suitable: in an era where women were struggling to look more like boys, it was fitting that one of their favorite blouse styles would be named after the boy who refused to grow up.

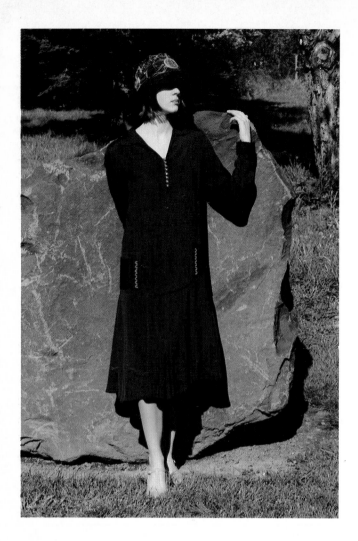

The "flapper look" most people think of when they think twenties. Made of navy crepe trimmed with bright orange buttons, this sort of dress is relatively easy to find today. *Courtesy of The Very Little Theatre.*

The most variety to be incorporated into blouses was in the sleeves. While kimono–style sleeves were favored for much of the decade, there was a seemingly endless assortment of other styles: fitted sleeves, "bell" sleeves (which were flared at the bottom), cap and cape–style sleeves, dolman and raglan sleeves, slit sleeves, and draped sleeves.

LINGERIE

"The pursuit of slimness is one of the chief labours of the modern woman," *Vogue* proclaimed in 1922—proving that while the Victorian corset was absolutely *passé*, the modern woman was just as concerned with her figure as her Victorian ancestor had been . . . the rules were just different. "With the aid of the corsetièr, the physical culturist, and the non–starchy diet, shall we soon develop a race of slender, willowy women?" asked *Vogue*. But a world of serpentine women never emerged.

The woman of the twenties was all–concerned with slimness, right from the start of the decade. In a sudden and rash move, fashion decreed that corsets were banished, leaving women who had relied on them for years with every bump revealed. "After being tolerated for a season or two," Carrie Hall wrote in her book of fashion reminisces, "this total unrestraint on a woman's figure went into oblivion. The *apparently* uncorseted figure was desirable, but the *absolutely* uncorseted mode was scoffed out of existence." Thus, the corset remained the most important article of clothing a woman owned.

Still, the new corset (now increasingly referred to as a "girdle") was a long way away from the rigid, heavily boned creature worn at the turn of the century. Though they were often still long (usually reaching the thigh), and often had two to four bones in the front (to help flatten the tummy), they were far more comfortable concoctions of elastic and rubber. "The flexible girdle," Nemo–flex said of their most modern corsets, "guiltless of back laces, has generous panels of the soft yet firm elastic webbing which does the holding in so much better and more gently than bones did...The joy of corsets that will hold your figure in without heavy boning is the magic of modern times!"

The second most important item every fashionable woman insisted upon owning was the "flattener" or "bandeaux." Though cupped bras wouldn't appear until 1928 (when, in general, curves began emerging), bandeaux were certainly forerunners of the bra. They began humbly, first as a boned chemise at the turn of the century, then evolving into a simple, straight tube made of strong cotton with narrow shoulder straps to support it. Occasionally, it had slight darts (which, like dresses of the era, ran *horizontally*, not vertically). Later in the decade, some were almost entirely made of elastic, and often attached to the girdle for an ultra-slim line. Ironically, though there was much talk about how "unkind" the wasp-waisted corset of the past had been to women's health, there were no complaints about the discomfort or unhealthiness of flattening the breasts.

Though in the early 1920s petticoats persisted in some circles (still being frilly, frothy little things), they gave way to simple, full-length slips by 1923. Another Victorian dinosaur—bloomers—also persisted through the first half of the decade. The bloomer of the twenties, however, ranged in length from mid-calf (under longer skirt) to above the knee, until, by 1927, bloomers (now more often called "knickers") ended at the top of the thigh. But the really modern way to wear "undies" (as they were now fashionably called) was to don a pair of "step-ins," which were, essentially, tap pants or panties. These usually ended at the top of the thigh, but could also end just above the knee.

Old–fashioned women still wore chemises, but combinations (Victorian–created garments that, true to their name, combined the chemise and the petticoat or bloomers) were more frequently worn. Appropriately, however, even combinations were modernized by shortening them to the top of the thigh and then re-dubbing them "Teddies." The new motto in lingerie was definitely "shorten, lighten, and stop the layering!"

Through most of the decade very simple lingerie was preferred, but it very often had crocheted trim or embroidered motifs (usually home-made)—a style that was inspired by the needle-arts revival that swept over the middle class during the decade. Needlework magazines also gave endless instructions for (and had much to do with the new–found popularity of) boudoir caps. In Victorian days they were dubbed, less glamorously, "night caps," but *boudoir* caps were all–new, and surprisingly ornate: crocheted, embroidered, and festooned with ribbons, embroidery, and nearly every type of trim imaginable. Perhaps this was the way women added just a dash of old–fashioned femininity to their wardrobe. Still, the modern woman strove to eliminate anything even remotely Victorian from her wardrobe, and soon gave the boot to white "undies"; she was discreet about this, however, and stuck to pastel shades.

Early in the decade, Paris decreed that the truly fashionable woman would wear no stockings—a clear revolt against hot, sticky stockings that had for generations pulled at every move. However, few women were brave enough to go bare legged, and instead adopted flesh–colored hose. Few other colors were manufactured, except for the traditional black. But a popular vaudeville joke of the time expressed how fashion felt about *that*: "Q: Whatever happened to the girl in the black stockings? A: Nothing." Flappers who wanted the protection of a stocking but wished to ditch the discomfort of garters, rolled their hose. When worn with short skirts, flappers revealed bare thigh and a wad of rolled hose at their knee. Less daring women chose decorative and often elaborate garters, knowing that, no matter how careful they were when they sat, their garters *would* be revealed.

Unfortunately, while the new rayon hose were far less expensive than silk stockings, they only added to the flapper's "thrown together" look, bagging and gathering miserably at the ankles. Still, unless a woman was willing to give in to the old–fashioned look of cotton stockings rayon was her only alternative to expensive silk. Then, in 1929, with a little coal, water, air, and vegetable oil, W.H. Carothers made a mistake while trying to make artificial rubber. This "mistake" ended up being the invention that set the lingerie industry on its ear, and within that same year, his newly–discovered "nylon" began appearing in almost every sort of lingerie—including (late in the 1930s) stockings.

When a woman wished to lounge around the house, she no longer did so in what her mother affectionately referred to as a "teagown," instead, she dawned a kimono or—better yet—pajamas. No, pajamas were not yet considered sleepwear, but, as *Vogue* stated in 1924, were now considered "by far the smartest form of négligée." Worn at the beach, around the house, or at casual, relaxed events dubbed "Pajama Parties," they provided ultimate comfort.

SPORTSWEAR

"Women cannot ride astride because most of them are not built that way..." *Vogue* warned in 1922. "If a woman insists upon riding like a man, please, oh, please let her consult a physician first." Though most Victorianisms were banished in the twenties, some prejudices and misunderstandings about women persisted. Nonetheless, few women rode side-saddle anymore, and the old riding habit of long, heavy, draped skirts was dead. The new riding habit—sleek, and very "modern"—was, in essence, the same English riding costume worn today: a simple, tailored jacket and a pair of full–thighed riding trousers. Yes, trousers!

In the past women who wore trousers (ordained solely as men's clothes) were thought to be as ridiculous as men who wore women's dresses. But in the 1920s, trousers were slowly becoming an acceptable woman's garment. They were, however, reserved for sporting: horseback-riding, hunting, fishing, and golfing.

Bathing suits had changed little by 1920, and were still surprisingly Victorian, consisting of a pair of bloomers worn under a rather full-skirted dress. By 1922, however, while Sears catalog offered mostly dress-like bathing suits, they did offer one suit that was thoroughly modern and looked remarkably like the suit Gertrude Ederle wore in 1926 when she became the first woman to swim the English Channel (beating the male record by a full two hours): one-piece, no skirt, clingy, short sleeves, with a scooping neckline.

The bathing suit took on new significance in the 1920s, as sunbathing became *the* fashionable pasttime (a suntan proving that the lady *must* be a lady of leisure). Beach life, suntans, and bathing suits were the new must for the fashionable woman—though swimming was never considered necessary. In fact, *Vogue* proclaimed in 1923, "whether to swim at all is a consideration, for swimming has a way of increasing girth in an amazingly short time." Later, the same magazine proclaimed: "The modern girl is triumphant. She can wear anything she wants to wear, but, if she is wise, she will be careful not to let her freedom go to her head. After all, a bathing suit tells a more honest story than any other form of dress." From longish-legged suits, to suits cut high on the hip, to sashed waistlines, to embroidered suits, to suits with decidedly weird color combinations, the woman of the twenties relished her newfound freedom—never any more pronounced than when she was on the beach.

Fancy Dress

Sadly, the twenties were the last act for fancy dress costumes. Though the tradition of masquerade balls and theatricals had thrived in the Victorian era, the tradition was slowly petering out. Still, twenties fancy dress costumes are easier to identify than those of earlier periods. No longer were lavish and abstract costumes favored (making them difficult to distinguish from "normal" evening wear); in the 1920s fancy dress often reflected the new commercialism of the era, copying figures such as the Quaker Oats man and the Ovaltine lady, clearly marking them as costumes. Kits and instructions abounded for making crepe paper costumes (though the crepe paper used then was much heavier and sturdier than today's). Sewing patterns for fancy dress were also still being produced (especially by the pattern giant Butterick), and well-sewn, well-planned costumes from the 1920s can still be found today.

Other Important Garments

The cloche hat is the hallmark of the 1920s—though wider brimmed, boat-like hats decorated with Victorian–style flowers were predominant before 1924. But it was the small, clingy, strikingly new cloche that women loved and nicknamed their "bobbed hats." In truth, however, even those who couldn't bear to bob their hair (which must have been an incredible act of bravery, since women had never before whacked off their "crowns of glory!") wore cloches by simply stuffing their tresses into cloches with high, full crowns.

Fans were still in use—but instead of the old-fashioned, dainty kind, the woman of the Twenties usually preferred a fan made up of one or two over-sized feathers, or a lavishly painted, oval-shaped or folding paper fan. Such paper fans frequently were "give-aways" and featured the artful advertising of perfumes, restaurants, and fashion. These are highly collectible—particularly if they are signed by a popular artist.

Though gloves were no longer thought necessary by most women, ladies of society coveted fine gloves with heavy decoration and wide, gauntlet-style cuffs. Parasols had their last stand in the 1920s. The new style was no longer frilly or fussy; most women preferred the Oriental paper type, especially at the beach.

Costume jewelry—once largely pooh-poohed—finally came into its own in the twenties, and compacts (though used somewhat in the 'teens) also finally "made it." Beaded bags, like beaded dresses, were *the* "thing." Other types of bags were certainly in use, however, including mesh bags and (especially for those women who needed to carry more than a hanky and change) leather handbags.

Other accessories, including decorative headbands and cigarette holders, were exceedingly popular among the fashionable set and have come to be thought of as the epitome of the Roaring Twenties; one less-remembered accessory, however, was the hip flask. From very plain to gemstone-encrusted, flasks were considered quite necessary by certain sets during Prohibition. Other items, such as hollow-headed canes, were also a direct reaction to the Volstead Act.

Shawls became works of art in the twenties. Lavishly embroidered and often fringed, these oversized piano shawls added an ethnic flavor and a relieving femininity to the otherwise angular fashions of the decade. Fur coats also added a softer edge to fashion, as did wrap-around cocoon coats in satins and brocades.

In the early part of the twenties, high-buttoned boots were still worn by many. However, as interest was increasingly given to rising hemlines, pumps, T-straps, and tailored-looking Oxford shoes were favored. It was also from a new "modern" way of wearing shoes that flappers got their name; as author Carrie Hall remembers it: "The flapper wore her galoshes unfastened, and they flapped to her heart's content."

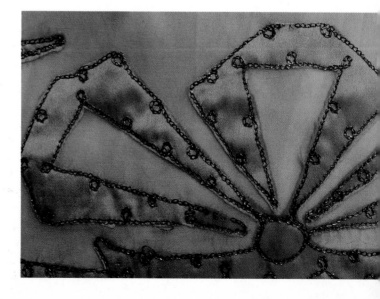

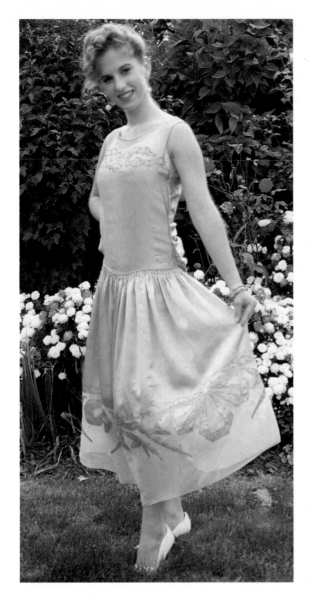

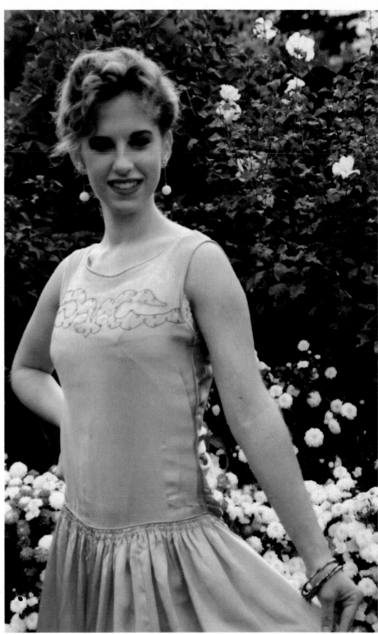

Slip-like dresses were the prominent style of the twenties. This satin and organza dress features unusually feminine appliqué embellishment.

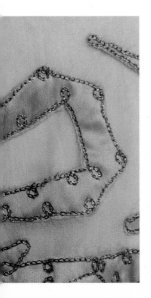

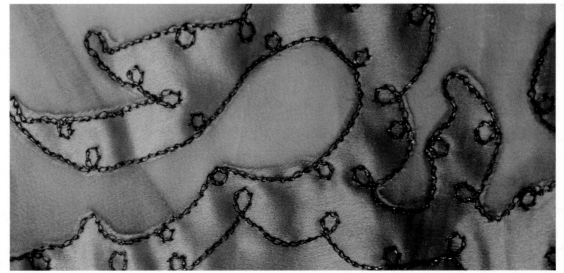

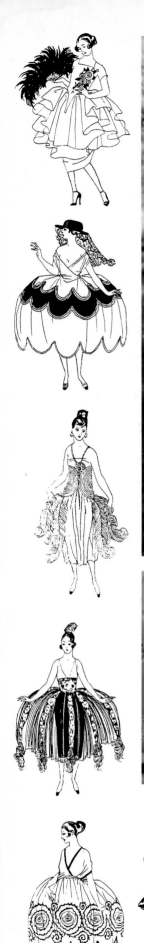

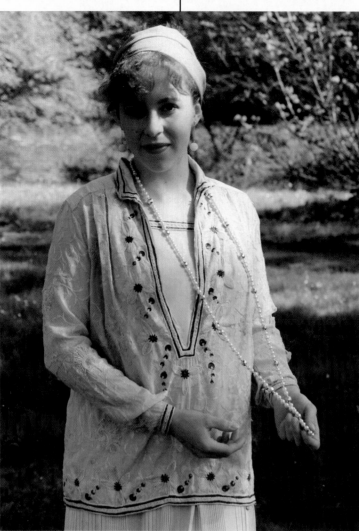

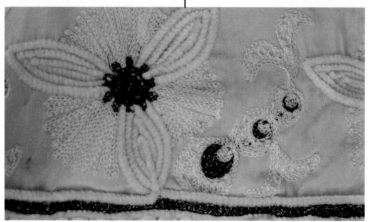

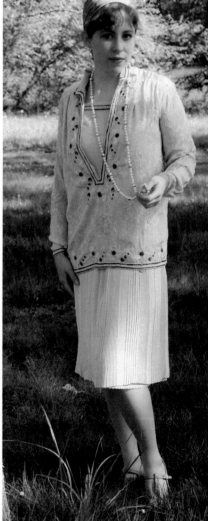

This ensemble—consisting of a tubular dress worn under an over-blouse—does not contain a couture designer label, but it almost certainly was made by one; it is entirely handstitched by skilled hands, and the embellishments are exquisite. *Courtesy of The Very Little Theatre.*

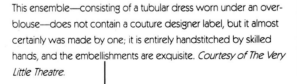

Though fashion magazines and fabric manufacturers pushed opulent styles like these in 1920, few women adopted them, and they are difficult to find today.

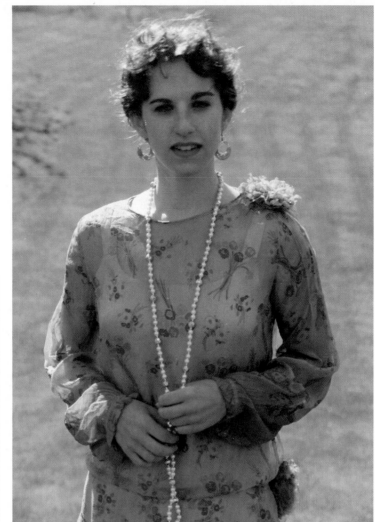

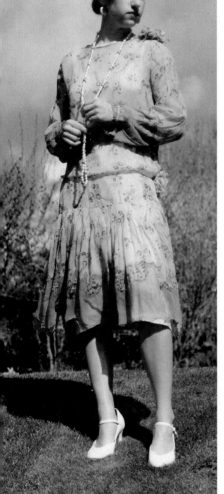

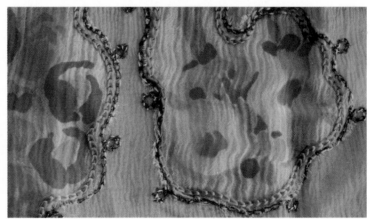

Made up in widely popular twenties colors, this chiffon dress is extremely well made, featuring fabric pom-pons at the shoulder and hip and carefully handfinished details. The skirt, which appears to be finished with a border print, it actually appliquéd. *Courtesy of The Very Little Theatre.*

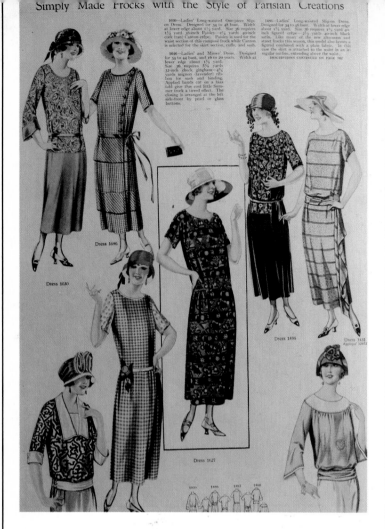

A *Pictorial Review* sewing pattern fashion plate from 1923. Though simple in comparison to early 1900s styles, the garments shown are still quite feminine.

An elegant dress designed by Worth and featured in *Gazette du Bon Ton* in 1922.

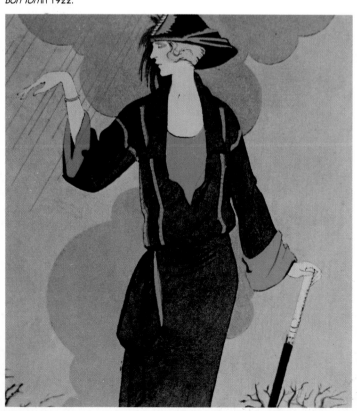

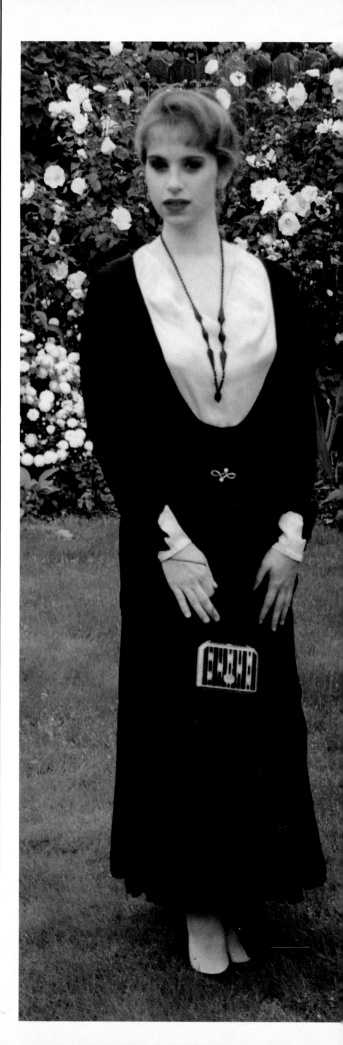

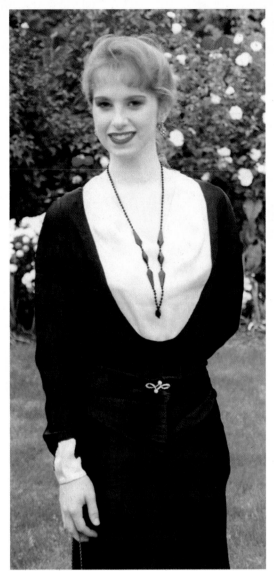

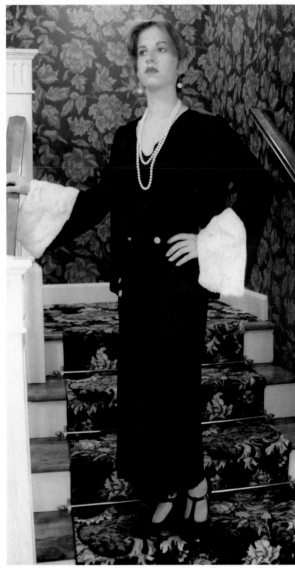

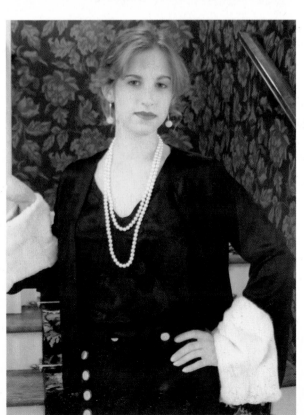

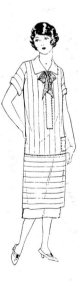

Previous Page and Above:
A black and ecru satin dress from the late twenties, featuring tiny pleats in the skirt. The "waistband" does not reach around the back of the dress, but begins at the sides, and is closed with a fashion pin. *Courtesy of The Very Little Theatre.*

Right and Above Right:
A three-piece suit featuring a satin blouse, a tubular silk skirt trimmed with buttons, and an easy-fitting silk jacket embellished with fur cuffs. *Courtesy of Persona Vintage Clothing.*

Far Right Illustration:
A simple, tailored dress, as featured in the Winter 1925 issue of *Every Woman Her Own Dressmaker.*

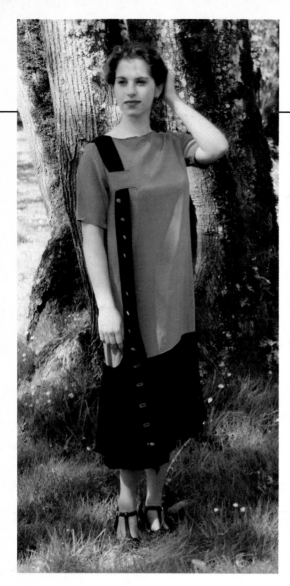

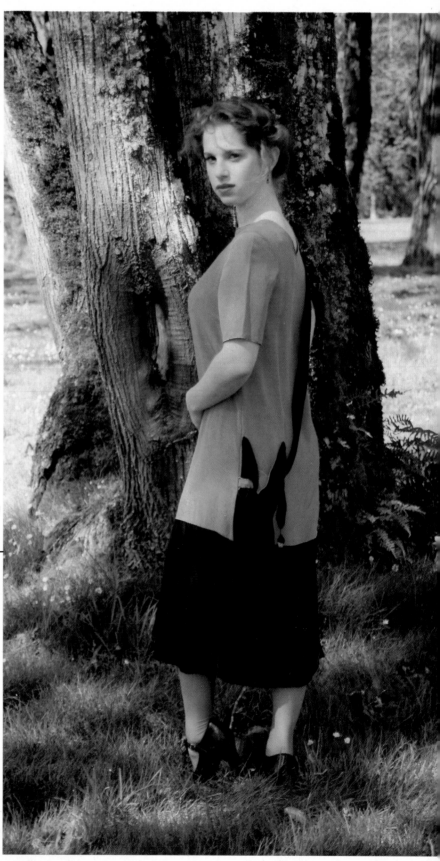

Though undeniably twenties, this little dress reveals at least one old-fashioned feature: "split-pin" buttons, which are pinned (not sewn) on, making it possible to remove and replace the buttons easily. *Courtesy of The Very Little Theatre.*

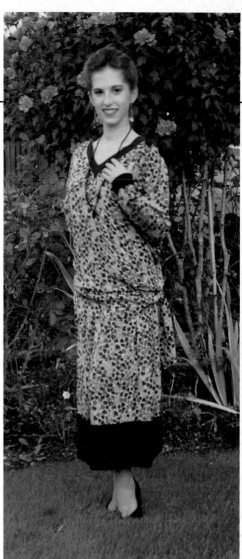

A brightly printed rayon dress, gathered lightly at the waist.
Courtesy of The Very Little Theatre.

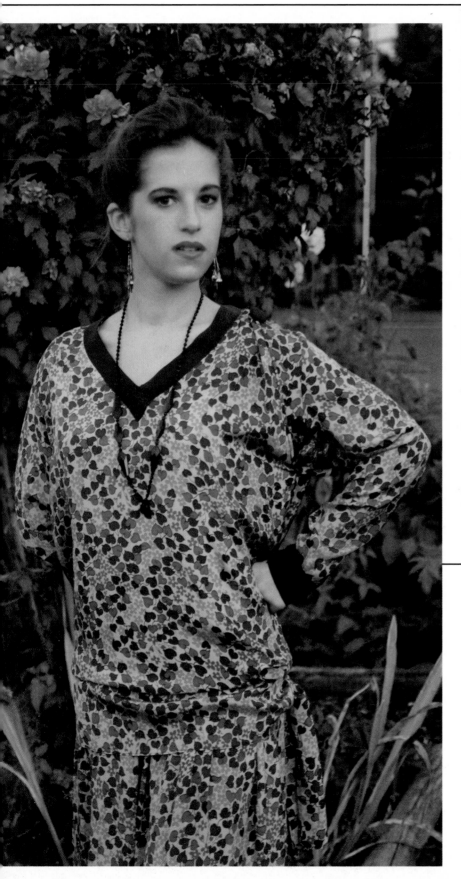

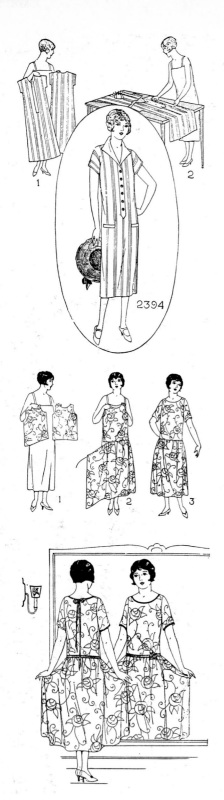

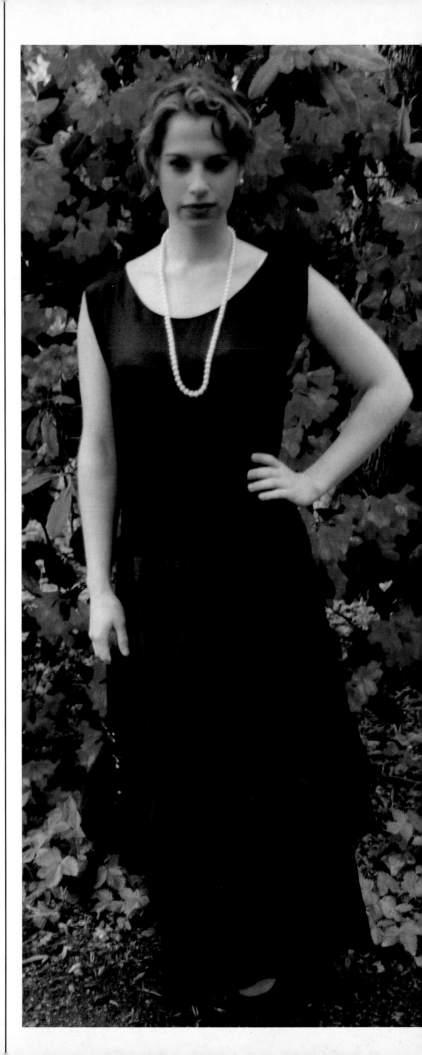

Because of clever marketing tactics, the home sewing industry really took off in the 1920s. Pattern companies frequently stressed that styles were easier to sew than ever before, but no one demonstrated this better than *The Fashion World*. In their catalog *Every Woman Her Own Dressmaker*, the simplicity of designs was clearly illustrated.

Late in the 1920s, flounces and longer hemlines appeared, foretelling the more feminine fashions of the 1930s. This dress is made up simply, in satin. *Courtesy of The Very Little Theatre.*

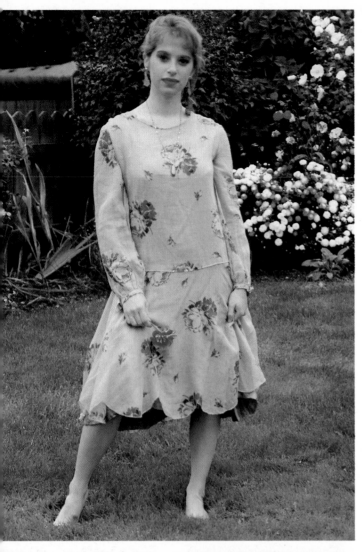

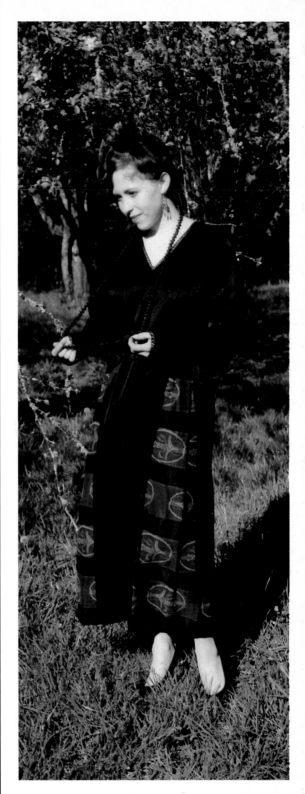

An elegant dress of black satin and panels of a woven, geometric design, circa 1920. *Courtesy of The Very Little Theatre.*

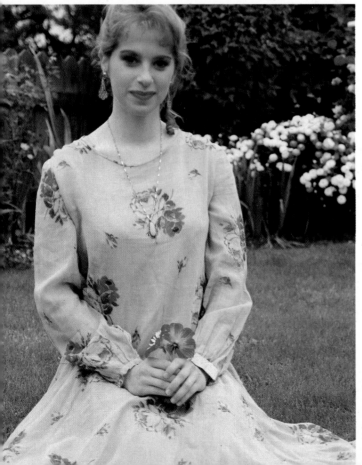

Breezy chiffon dresses were often favored in the twenties, but are difficult to find in good condition today. This one features a soft floral print, scalloped hemline, and a matching rayon underslip. *Courtesy of The Very Little Theatre.*

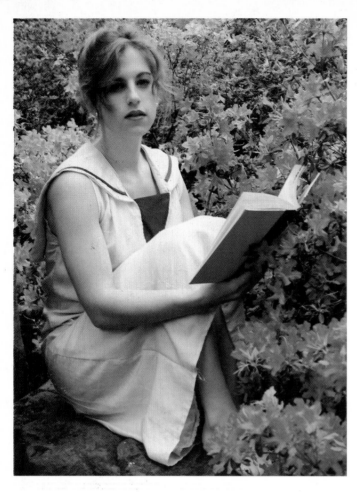

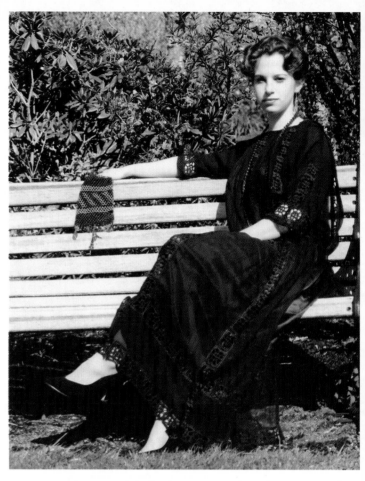

Sailor-style dresses and blouses were popular amongst young ladies in the twenties. This one is made of sturdy ecru and navy cotton, trimmed with navy braid. *Courtesy of The Very Little Theatre.*

A circa 1920 chocolate-brown chiffon dress featuring heavy lace inserts. *Courtesy of The Very Little Theatre.*

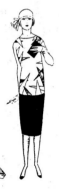

These simple dresses from 1925 illustrate clear use of Art Deco inspiration.

"Inspired By Things Oriental," from *The Pictorial Review*, 1923. Fabrics with Oriental influence were fashionable throughout the 1920s.

Following Page:
A circa 1920 afternoon dress of chiffon and lace with an attached underslip. *Courtesy of The Very Little Theatre.*

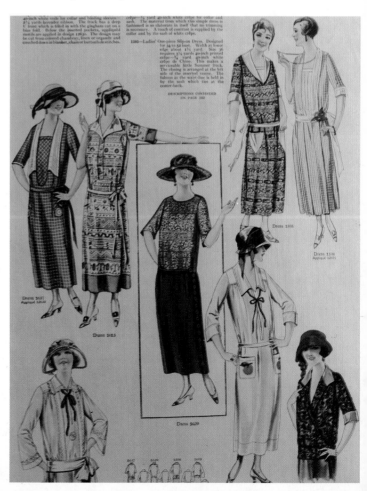

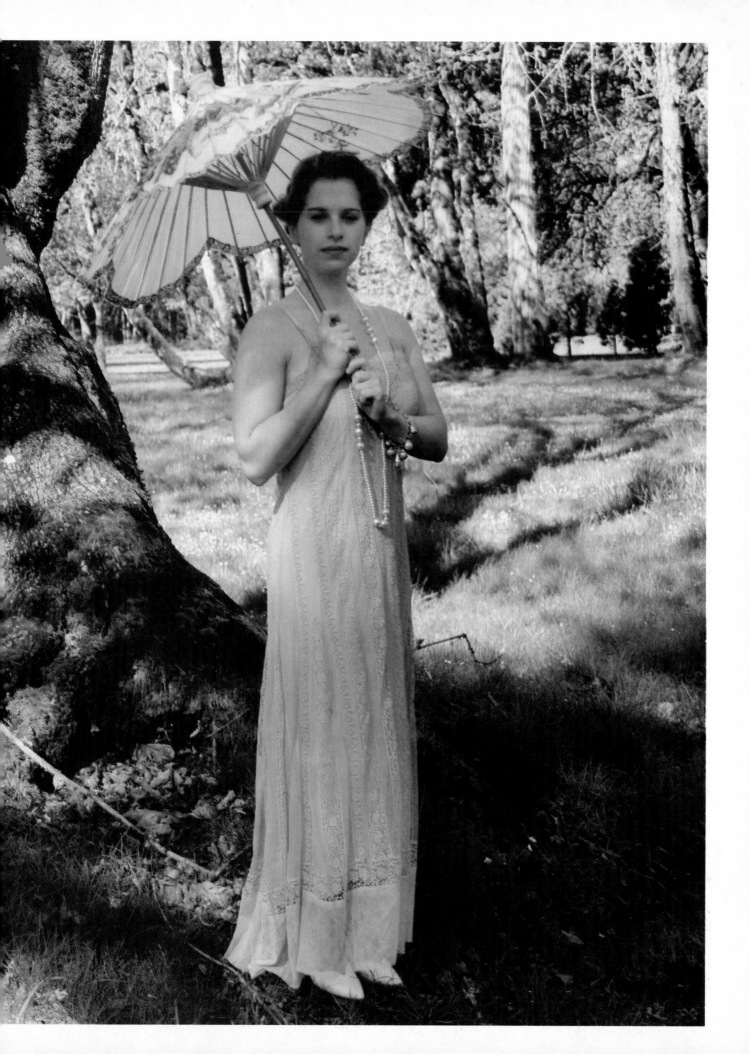

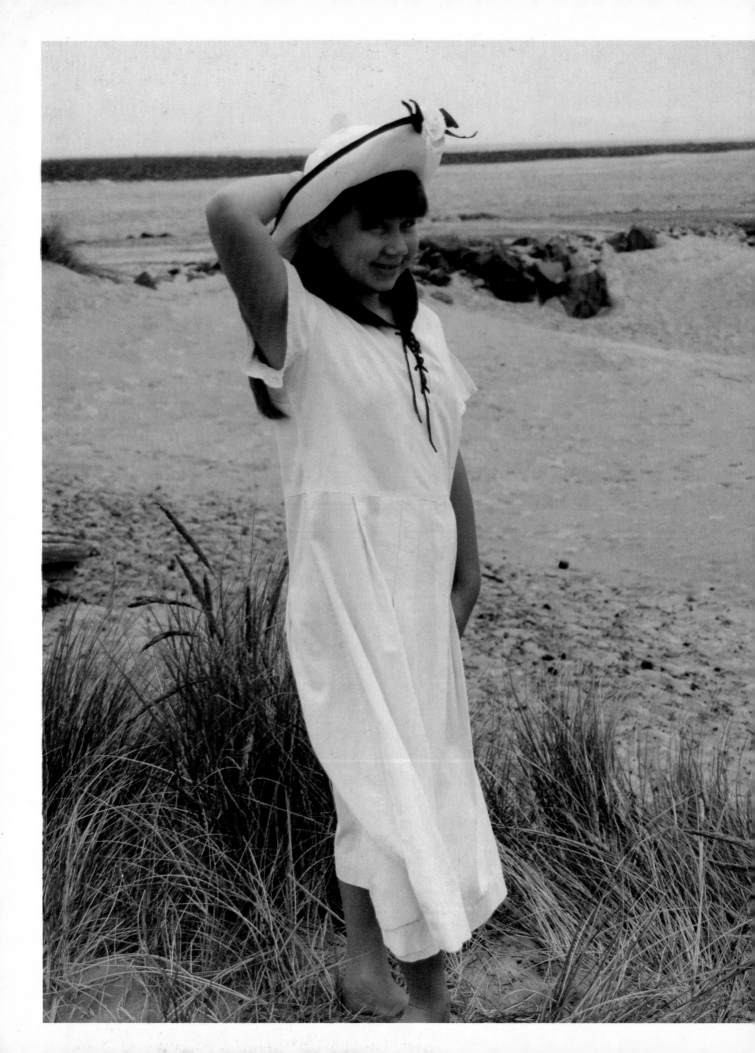

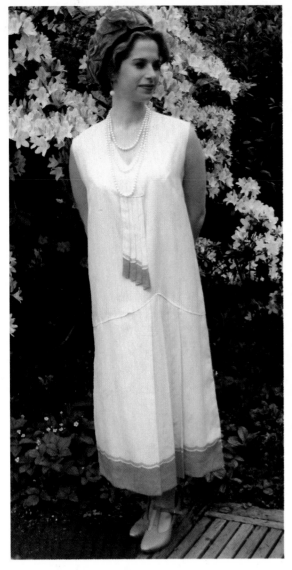

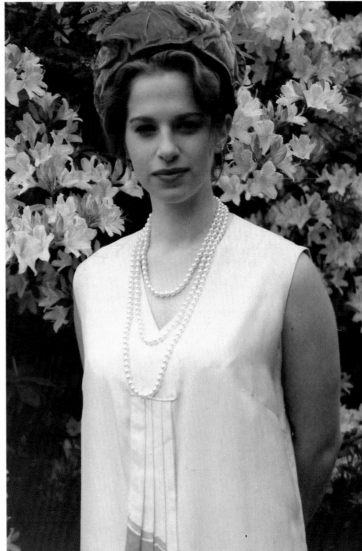

A classic 1920s day dress featuring a partially pleated skirt, a jabot, and a bold border print. Also notice the horizontal (slightly rising) darts in the bodice. *Courtesy of The Very Little Theatre.*

A chiffon dress with a matching slip, featuring flounces set in a saw-tooth line. *Courtesy of The Very Little Theatre.*

Previous Page:
This sailor-dress is of finer white cotton, and has no fastenings, save the lacing at the neckline. *Courtesy of The Very Little Theatre.*

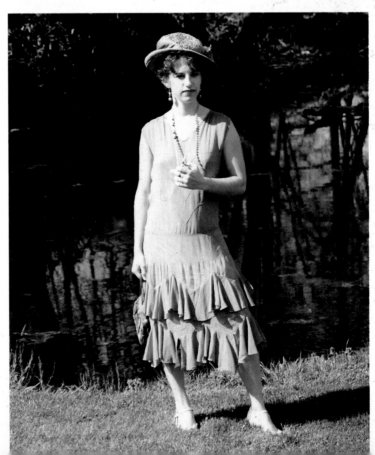

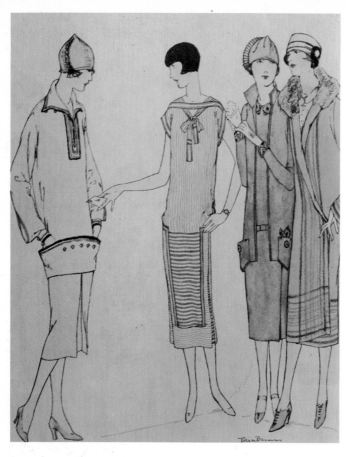

Tailored, angular styles "for business women," as featured in a 1925 issue of *Ladies' Home Journal*.

Three "everyday" styles as featured in *La Vie Parisienne* in 1922.

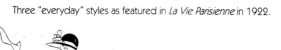

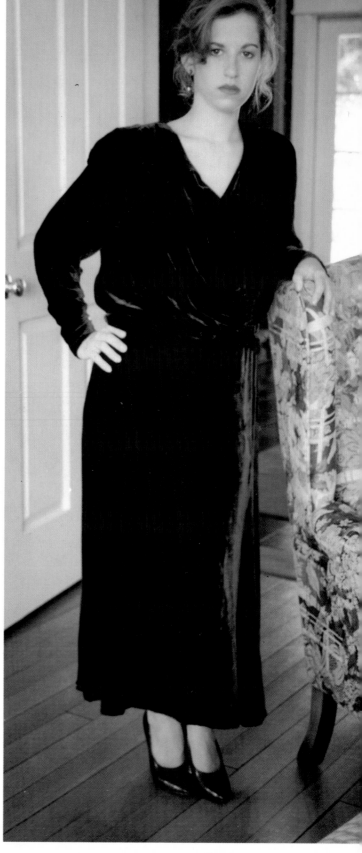

A supple, rich brown velvet dress. *Courtesy of Marianine's Vintage Chic.*

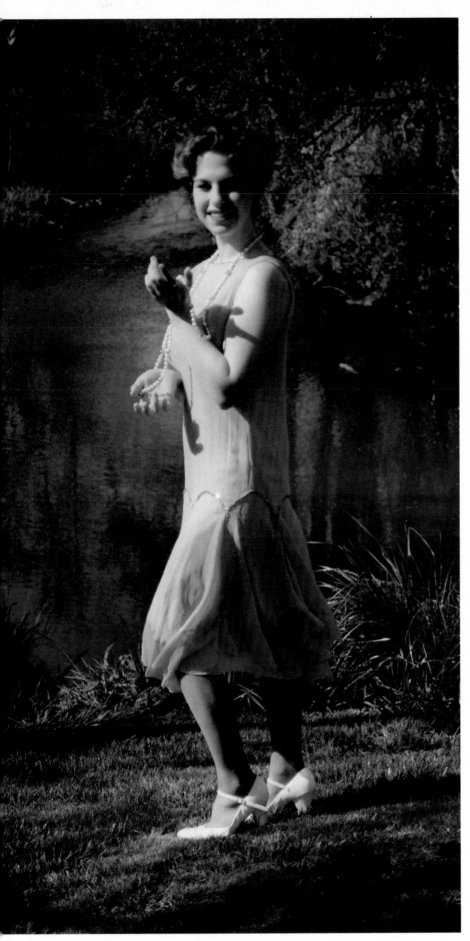

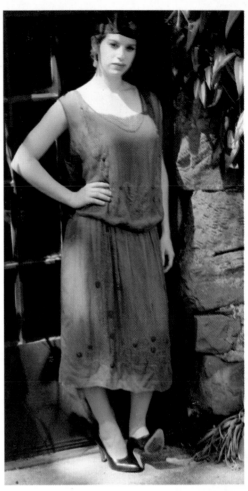

An unusual dress of brown chiffon beaded with brown and turquoise beads, and a colorful attached turquoise underslip. *Courtesy of The Very Little Theatre.*

A typical chiffon dress—made of rayon, which is more durable than silk, and therefore more frequently found today. *Courtesy of The Very Little Theatre.*

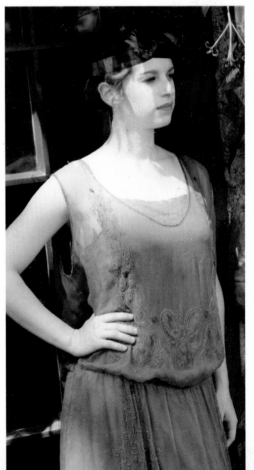

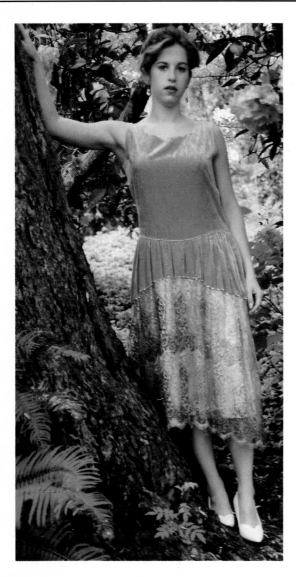

Of velvet, satin, and gold-shot lace, this dress, like many dresses of the period, has only three hooks and eyes (at a side seam) as closure. *Courtesy of The Very Little Theatre.*

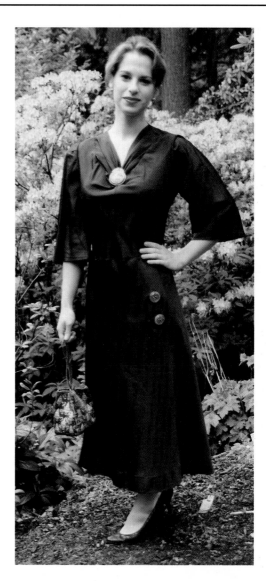

An unusual coat-style dress featuring a slight cowl neckline. *Courtesy of The Very Little Theatre.*

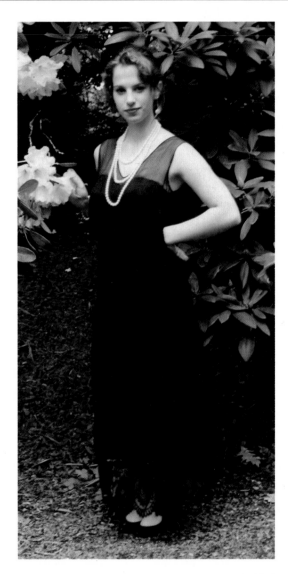

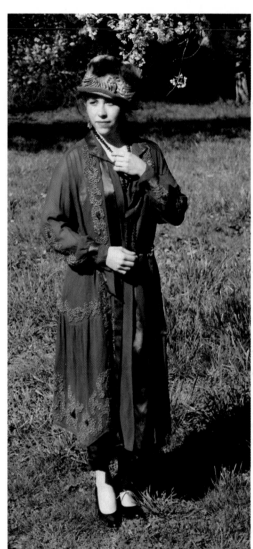

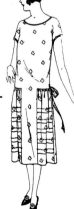

This simple dress of black chiffon, a satin underslip, and a black lace skirt slips over the head with no fastenings. *Courtesy of The Very Little Theatre.*

An elaborate dress (for the era, at least) made up of fine silk chiffon and lace. *Courtesy of The Very Little Theatre.*

A decidedly simple dress trimmed only with horizontal tucks.

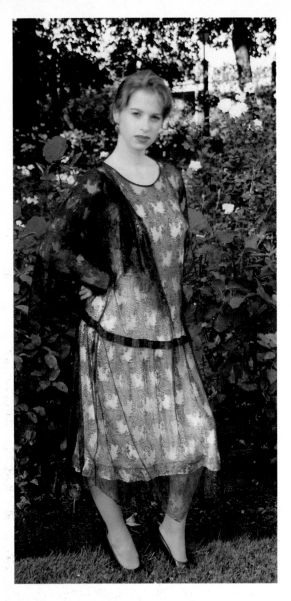

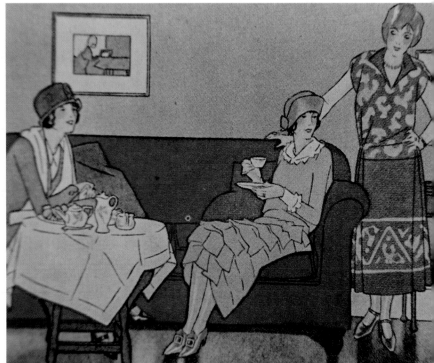

A silk lace dress featuring an uneven hemline, and wide, flowing sleeves. *Courtesy of Persona Vintage Clothing.*

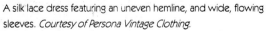

Three ladies as depicted in a 1925 advertisement. Notice the geometric print on the far right dress and the precise tucks on the dress in the middle.

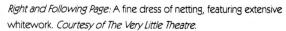

Right and Following Page: A fine dress of netting, featuring extensive whitework. *Courtesy of The Very Little Theatre.*

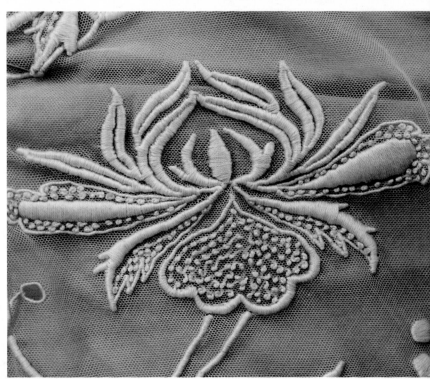

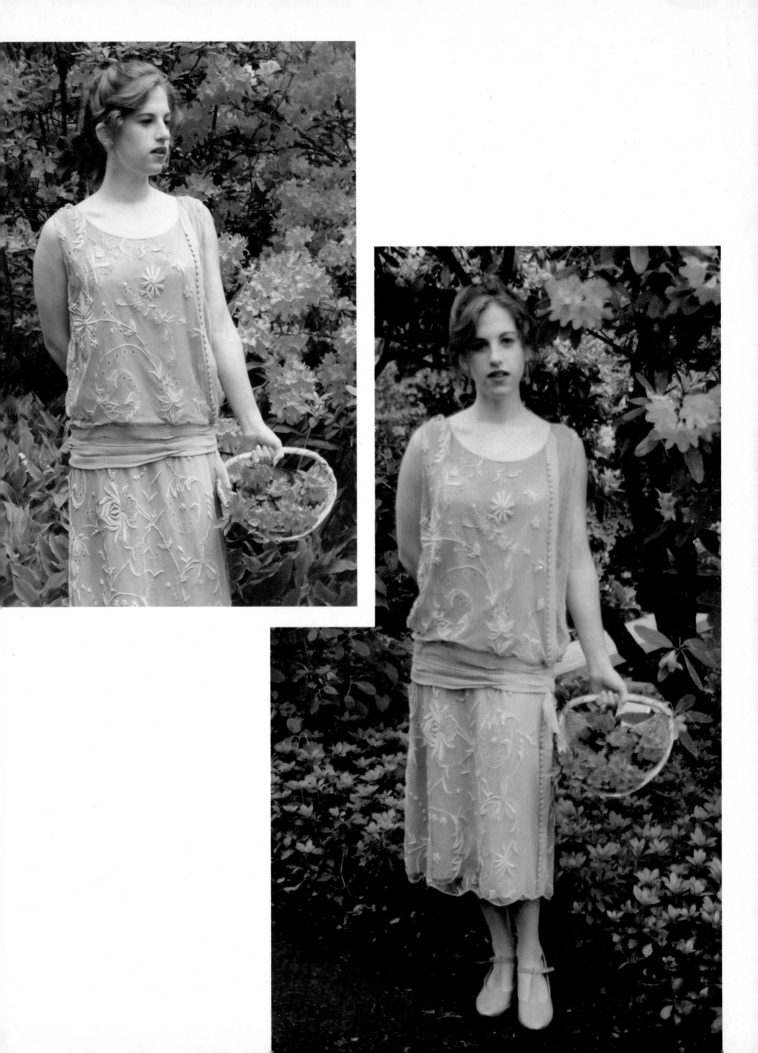

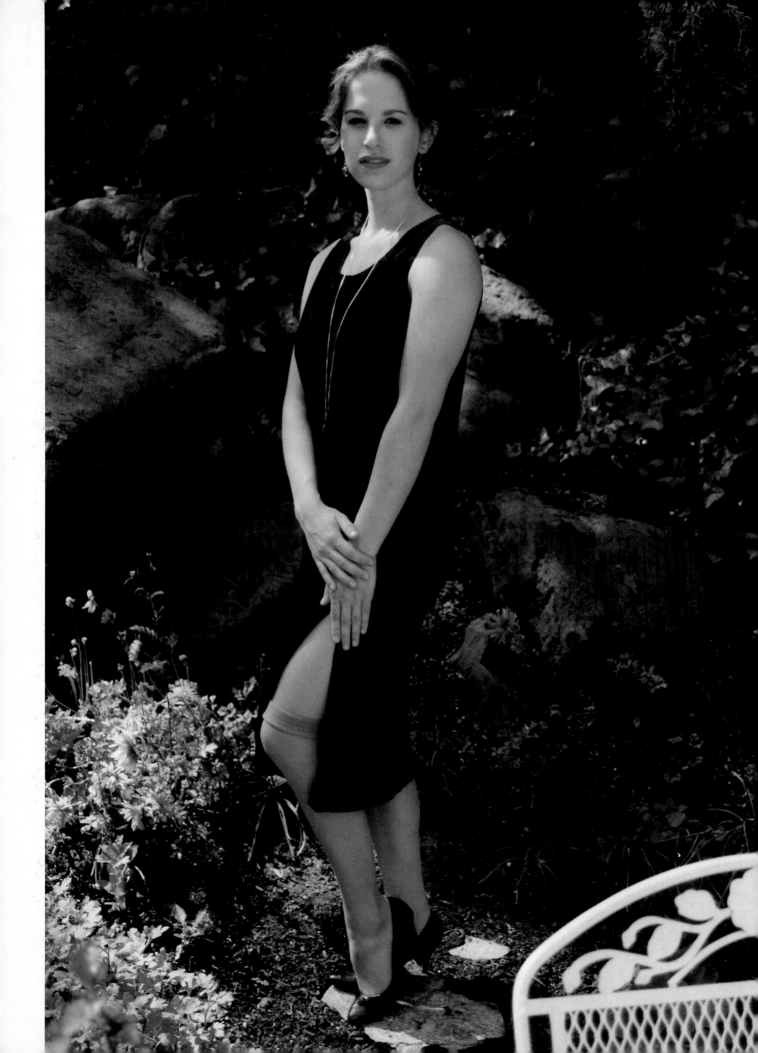

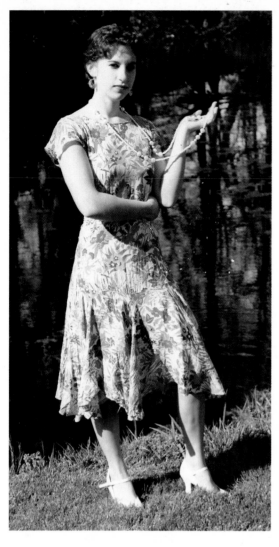

A wildly printed rayon dress, showcasing very short cap sleeves and an uneven hemline. *Courtesy of The Very Little Theatre.*

Previous Page:
A midnight blue velvet chemise dress of a very dark paisley design. *Courtesy of The Very Little Theatre.*

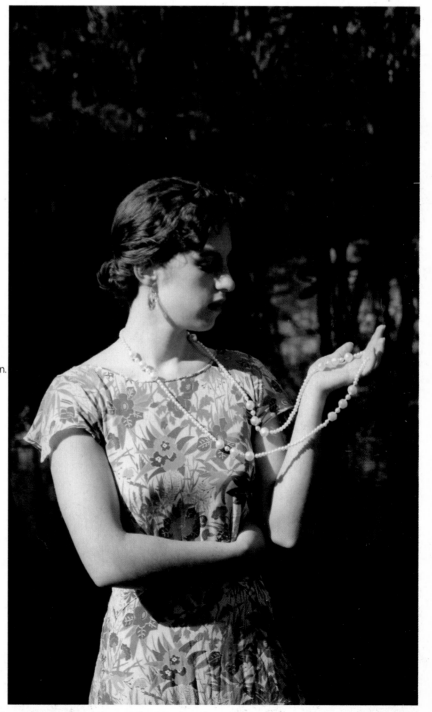

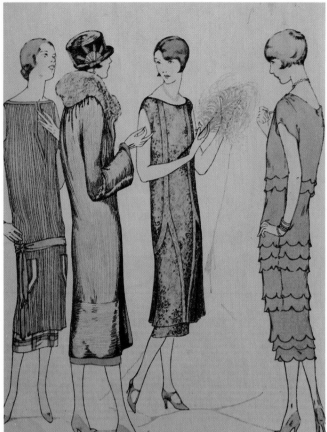

Dress designs as featured in *Ladies' Home Journal* in 1925.

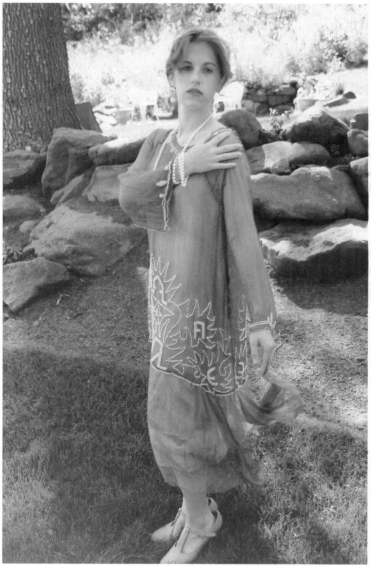

This chiffon dress features fine white beads with Egyptian-inspired motifs. *Courtesy of The Very Little Theatre.*

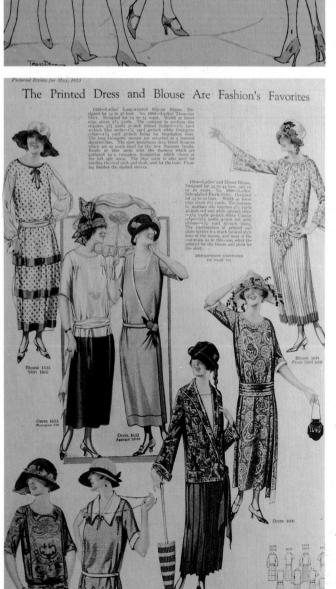

Following Page:
A sophisticated ensemble consisting of a silk chemise dress and a jacket of chiffon and marabou feathers. *Courtesy of Persona Vintage Clothing.*

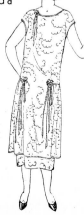

A 1925 sewing pattern sketch detailing a feminine day dress.

A 1923 sewing pattern fashion plate.

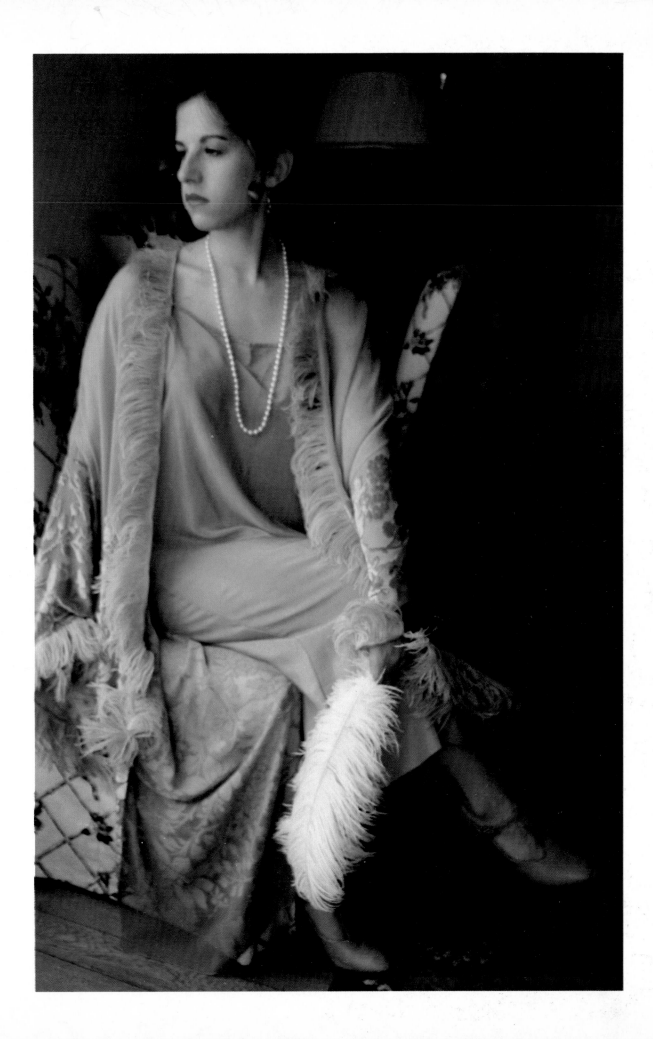

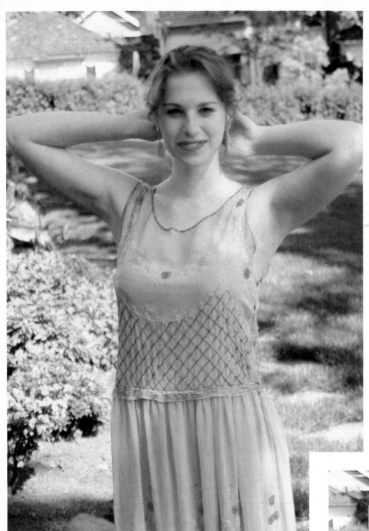

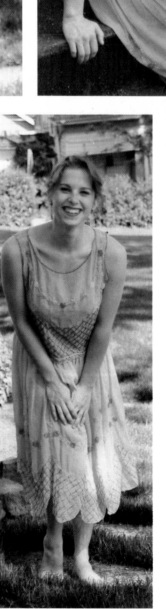

An exceptional chiffon beaded dress with a scalloped hemline, and mint, pink, rose, and yellow beads. *Courtesy of The Very Little Theatre.*

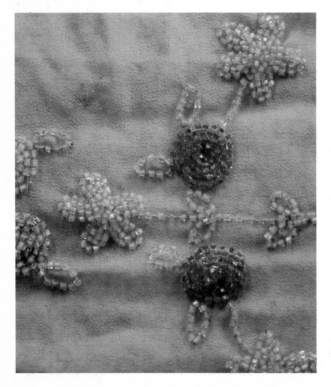

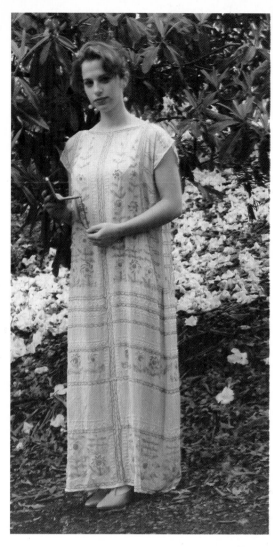

This full and concealing dress may have been worn during pregnancy. It features extremely detailed beading, and weighs nearly five pounds! *Courtesy of The Very Little Theatre.*

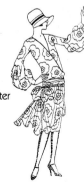

Toward the end of the decade, slightly softer styles were favored—like this one from a 1928 Parisian magazine.

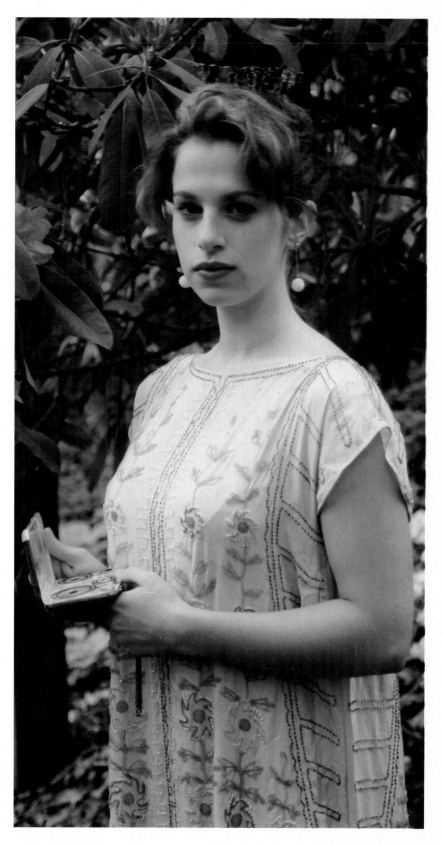

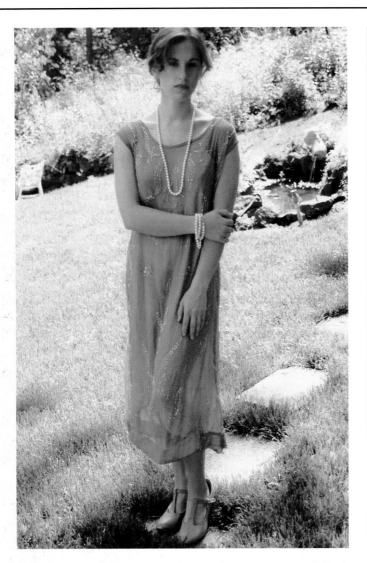

A exceptionally sheer chiffon dress featuring white beading.
Courtesy of The Very Little Theatre.

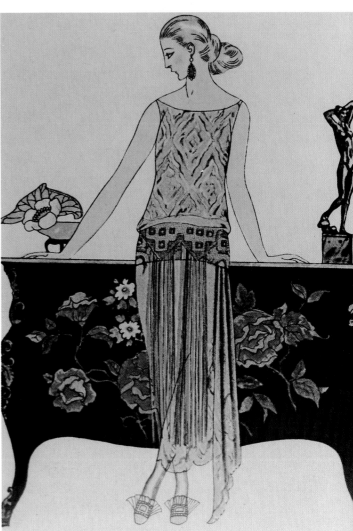

A 1922 couture evening gown by Worth.

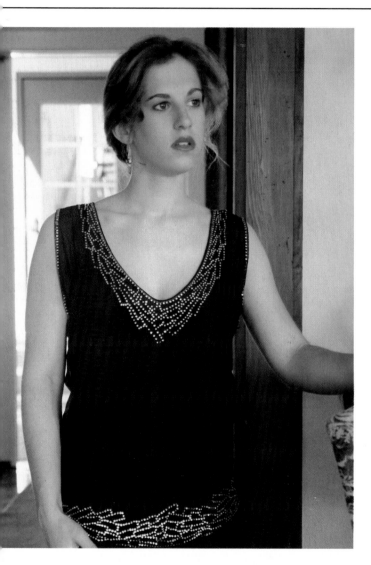

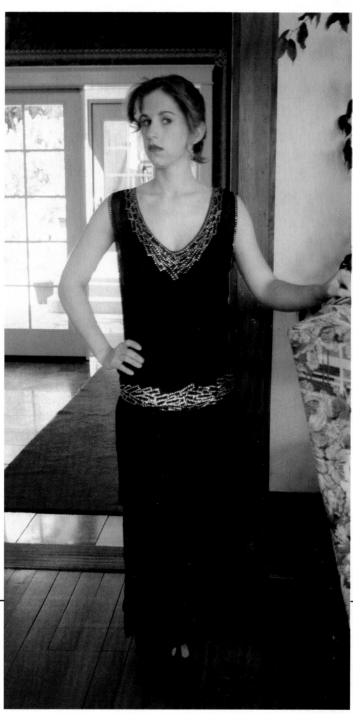

Though otherwise quite simple, this evening dress is made stunning by the use of Art Deco–styled rhinestones. *Courtesy of Sharon Jones.*

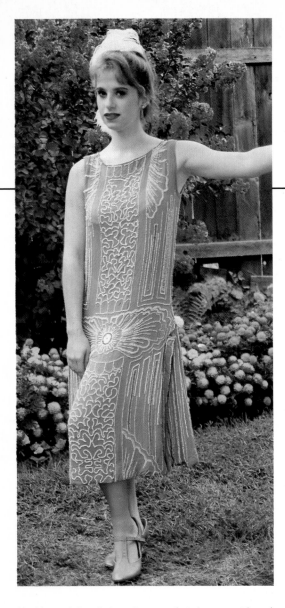

An elaborately beaded evening gown featuring geometric and Egyptian motifs.

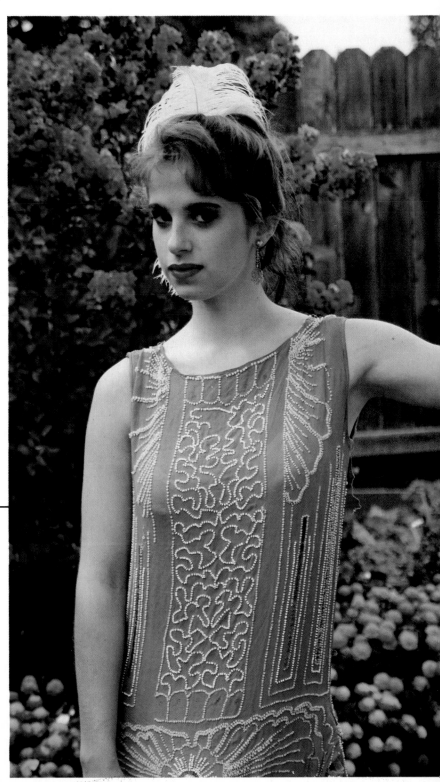

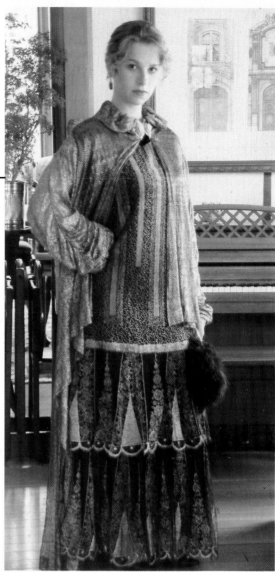

This dazzling gold-shot evening ensemble originally belonged to a vaudeville performer. The chemise-style dress hangs straight from the shoulder, but features flounces in the skirt. The jacket is as long as the dress, and is clasped only at the neck with an attached decorative buckle. *Courtesy of Persona Vintage Clothing.*

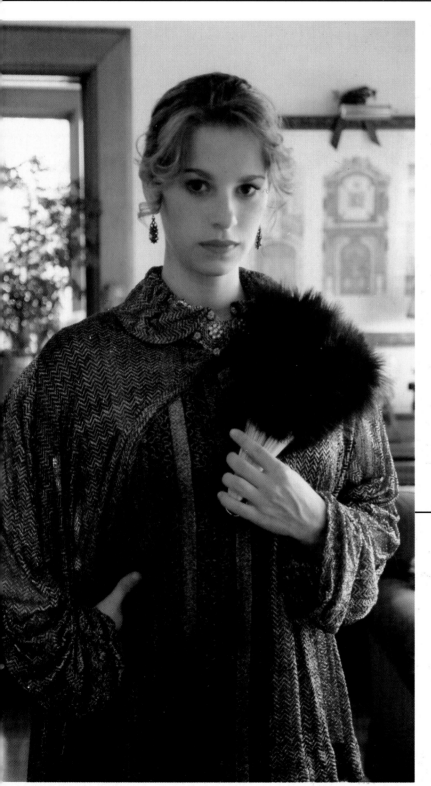

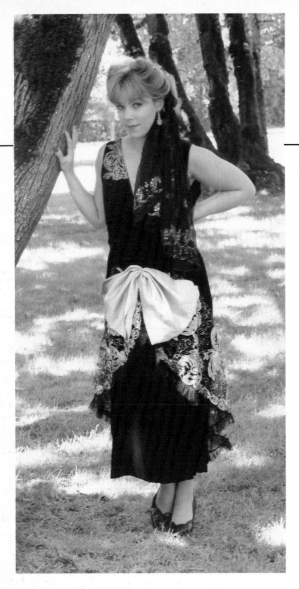

This Spanish-inspired, bohemian-style black chiffon and lace dress is shot with gold-metallics. *Courtesy of The Very Little Theatre.*

Long-line, over the hip blouses like these were favored for most of the twenties.

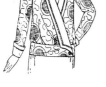

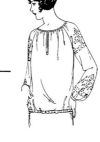

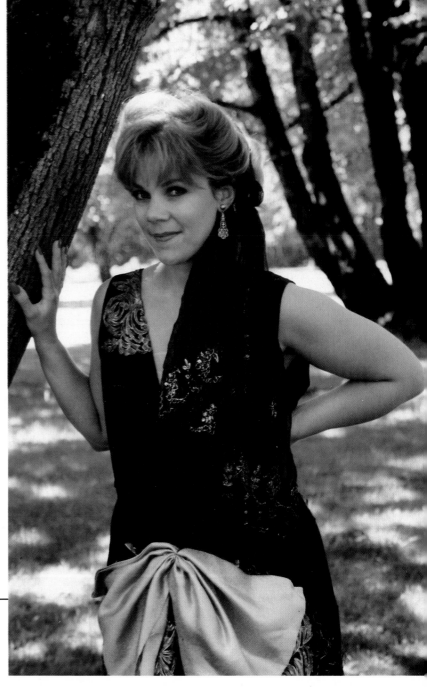

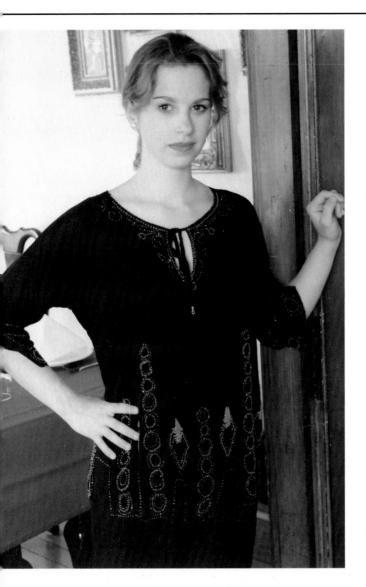

Once again, simple cut is made distinctive by the use of beaded trim and an uneven hemline. *Courtesy of The Very Little Theatre.*

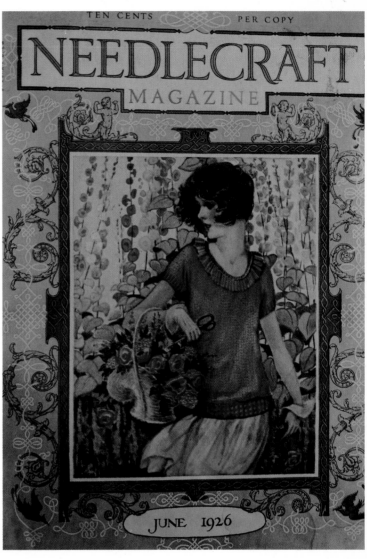

Needlework magazine frequently featured designs for creating sweaters.

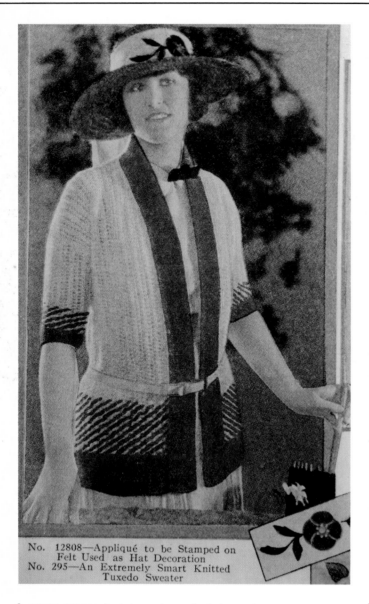

No. 12808—Appliqué to be Stamped on
Felt Used as Hat Decoration
No. 295—An Extremely Smart Knitted
Tuxedo Sweater

Sweaters were popular during cooler months, but were always
very simple.

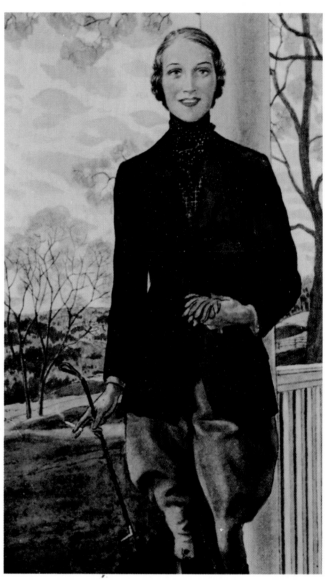

The "new and modern" riding habit, as featured in a period
advertisement.

A pants outfit featured in a 1920 issue of *La Vie Parisienne*. Such
outfits were hardly what the average woman cared to wear.

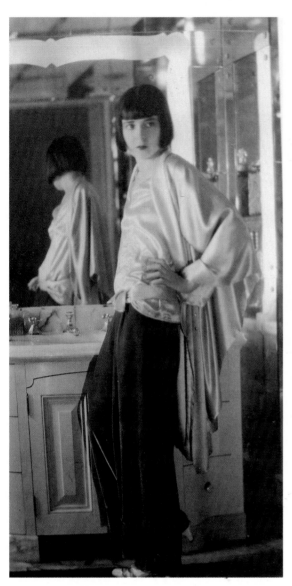

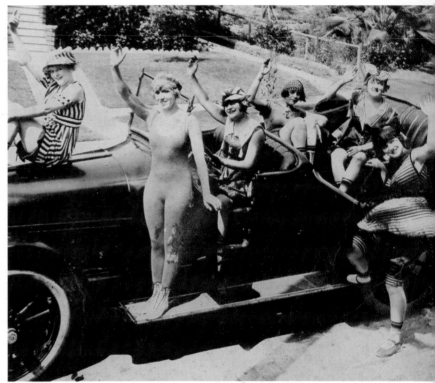

A frolicking group of young flappers dressed in some of the most revealing bathing suits seen in the decade. The girl second from the left wears a long, one-piece suit similar to that worn by champion swimmer Gertrude Ederle.

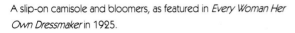

A more realistic view of the sort of pants women of the twenties chose to wear, modeled by Hollywood jazz baby Colleen Moore.

Undergarments, too, were decidedly simple to sew, as illustrated here by *Every Woman Her Own Dressmaker.*

A slip-on camisole and bloomers, as featured in *Every Woman Her Own Dressmaker* in 1925.

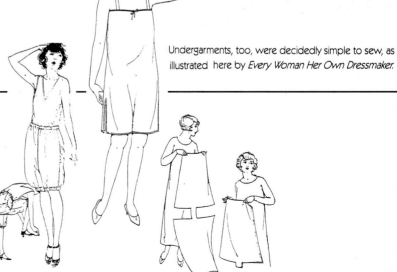

A 1925 Treo brand girdle. Their advertisement elaborates: "Treo Fashions are all made of surgical elastic webbing . . . combined with various brocade materials which encourage reducing and give the gracefully restricted figure with fashionable freedom."

A variety of Nemo-flex brand girdles and bandeaux.

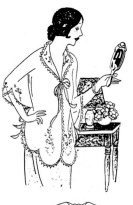

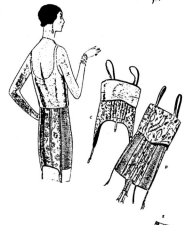

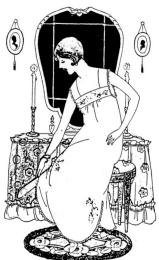

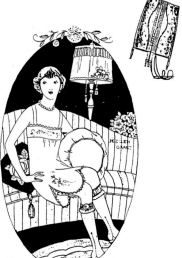

Needlework magazines regularly featured instructions for making embellished lingerie. These designs from *Needlecraft* illustrate a short slip and garters, a nightgown, and a short negligee or bed-jacket.

A boldly printed bathing suit featuring short knickers and a head scarf.

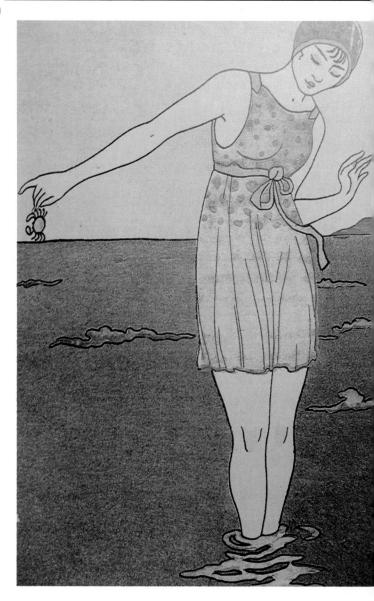

Though this Parisian fashion plate is dated 1913, it illustrates the sort of bathing attire many women would have worn in the early 1920s.

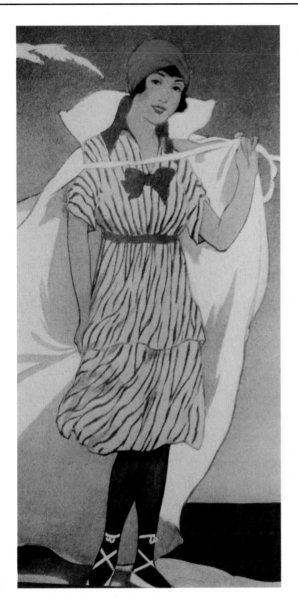

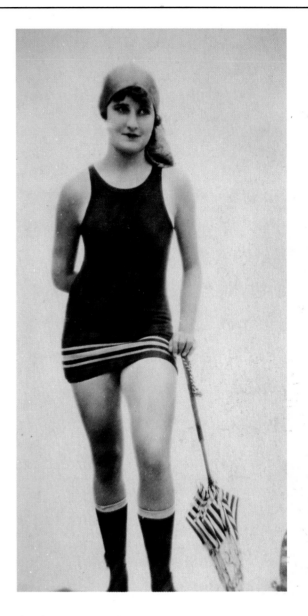

A circa 1919 bathing suit. Relatively full-skirted and simple, many women wore such suits well into the 1920s.

Though lean, simplistic suits were worn by many from around 1924 forward, old-fashioned bathing caps, stockings, shoes, and parasols were still toted to the beach.

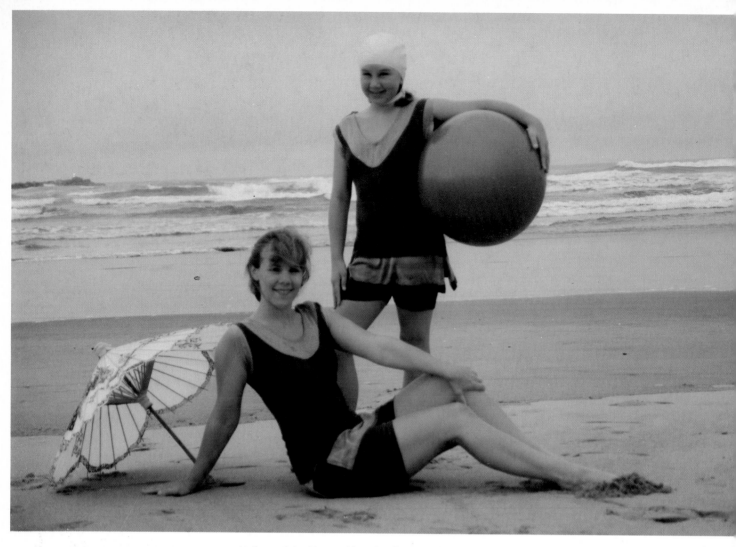

Mother and daughter matching suits. *Courtesy of The Very Little Theatre.*

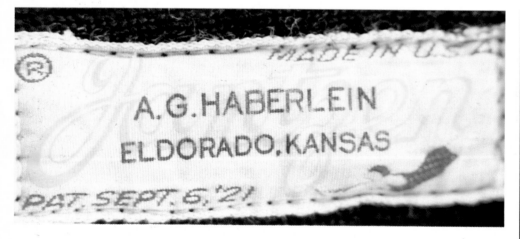

A.G. HABERLEIN
ELDORADO, KANSAS
PAT. SEPT. 6, '21

A nearly bare-backed suit featuring Jantzen's diving girl appliqué. The label indicates a patent date of 1921, but the suit may have first been sold a year or so after this time. *Courtesy of The Very Little Theatre.*

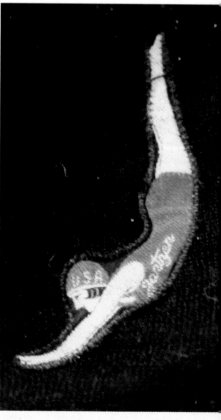

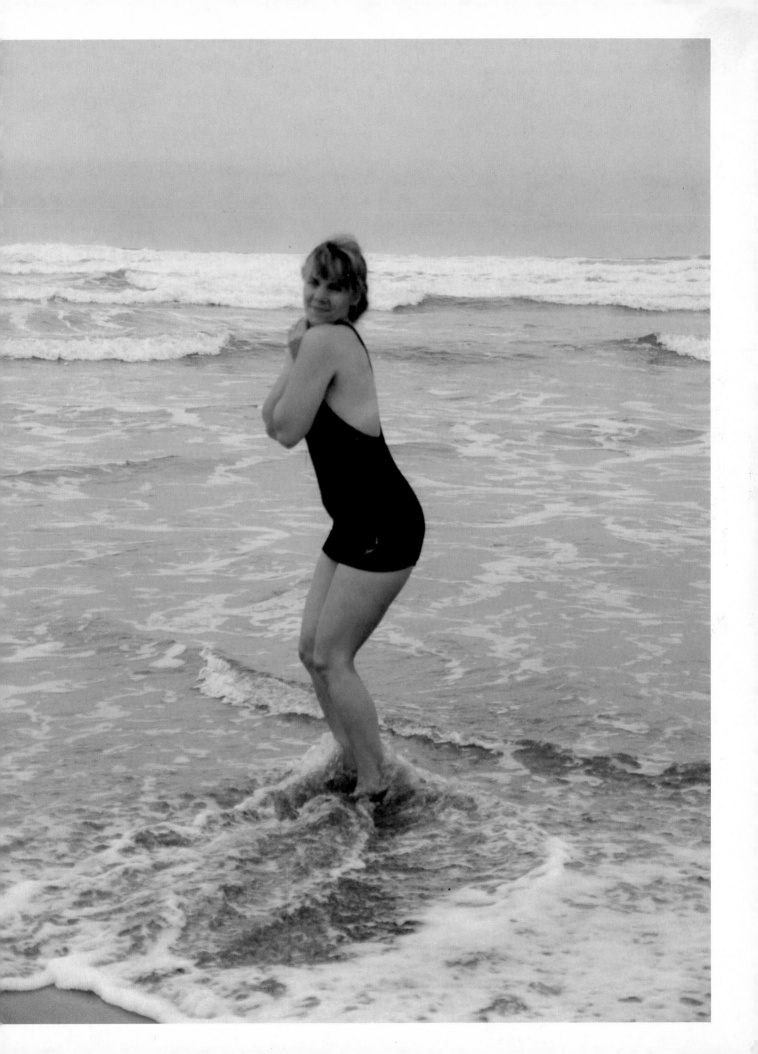

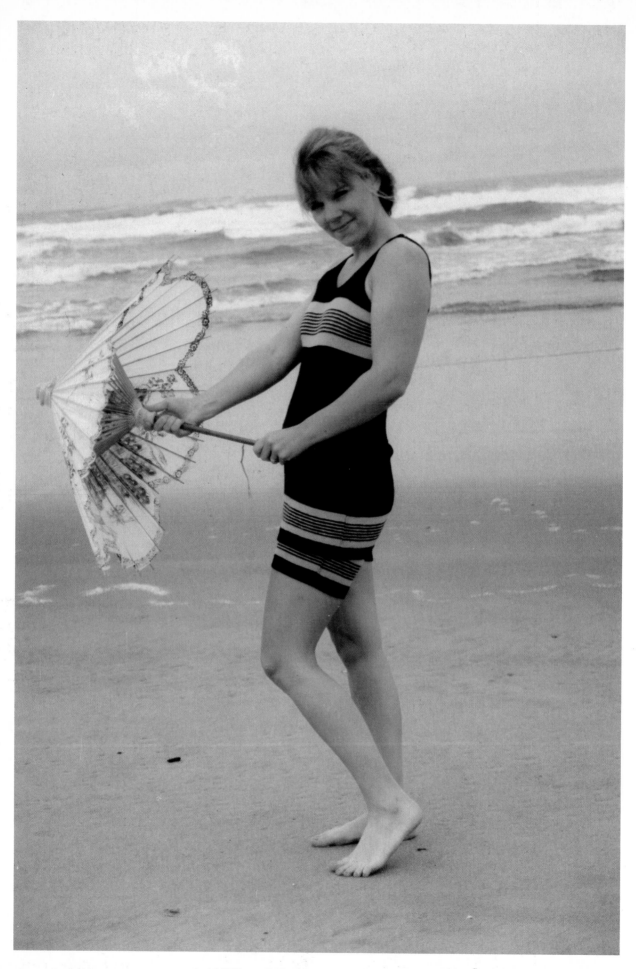

A mid-1920s wool suit. *Courtesy of The Very Little Theatre.*

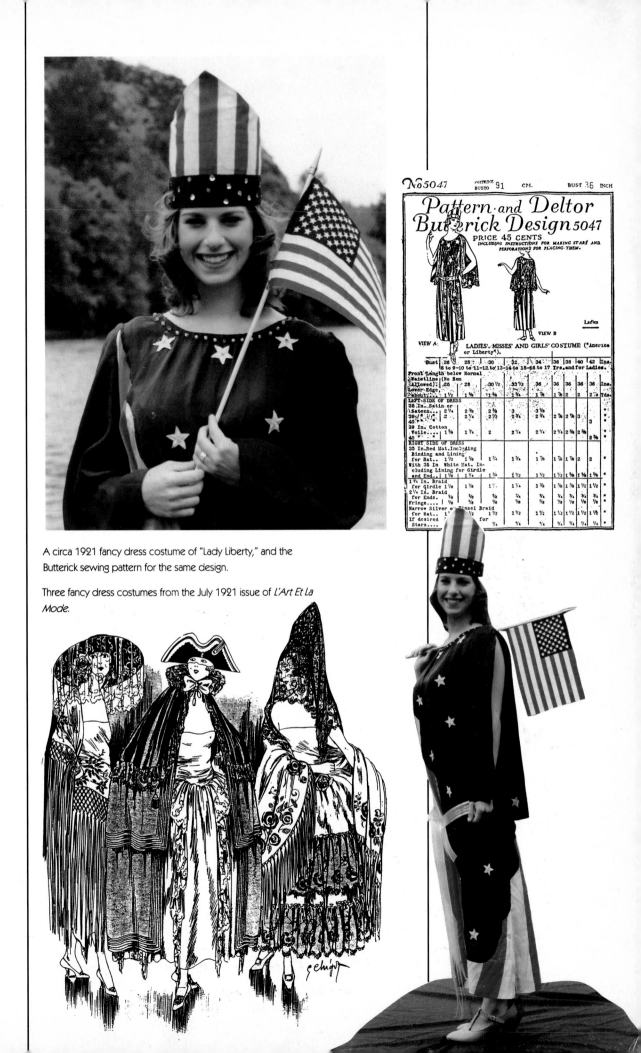

A circa 1921 fancy dress costume of "Lady Liberty," and the Butterick sewing pattern for the same design.

Three fancy dress costumes from the July 1921 issue of *L'Art Et La Mode.*

No.5047 PATTERN BUSTO 91 CM. BUST 36 INCH

Pattern and Deltor Butterick Design 5047
PRICE 45 CENTS
INCLUDING INSTRUCTIONS FOR MAKING STARS AND PERFORATIONS FOR PLACING THEM.

VIEW A VIEW B

LADIES', MISSES' AND GIRLS' COSTUME ("America or Liberty").

Bust	26	28	30	32	34	36	38	40	42 Ins.
	8 to 9	10 to 11	12 to 13	14 to 15	16 to 17 Yrs. and for Ladies.				
Front Length below Normal Waistline (No Hem Allowed)½	.25	.28	.30½	33½	36	36	36	36	Ins.
Lower-Edge, about....	1½	1⅝	1¼	¾	1⅞	1⅞	2	2	2⅛ Yds.
LEFT-SIDE OF DRESS									
35 In. Satin or Sateen....	2¼	2⅜	2½	3	3½				
39 ".	2	2¼	2½	2¾	2¾	2⅜	2⅞	3	
40 "								3	
39 In. Cotton Voile....	1⅝	1¾	2	2¼	2¼	2¼	2⅜	2⅜	
40 "									2¾
RIGHT SIDE OF DRESS									
35 In.Red Mat.Including Binding and Lining for Hat..	1½	1⅝	1¾	1¾	1⅞	1⅞	1⅞	2	2
With 35 In White Mat. Including Lining for Girdle and End..	1⅛	1¼	1¾	1½	1½	1½	1⅝	1⅝	1⅝
1¾ In. Braid for Girdle	1⅛	1⅛	1"	1¼	1¾	1⅜	1⅜	1½	1½
2¼ In. Braid for Ends..	⅜	⅝	⅝	¾	¾	¾	¾	¾	¾
Fringe....	⅛	⅛	⅛	⅛	⅛	⅛	⅛	⅛	⅛
Narrow Silver or Tinsel Braid for Hat..	1"	½	1½	1½	1½	1½	1½	1½	1½
If desired for Stars....			¼	¼	¼	¼	¼	¼	¼

Ladies

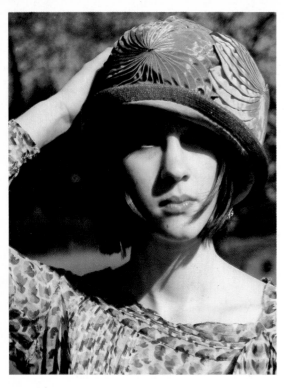

A typical hat, featuring bands of pleated silk. *Courtesy of The Very Little Theatre.*

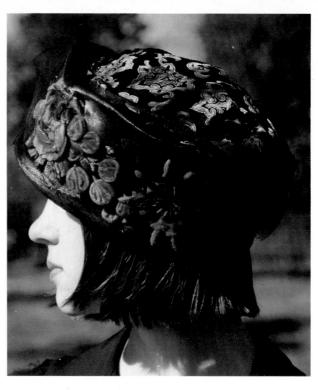

A frivolous and feminine hat, featuring gold-shot metallics and velvet flowers. *Courtesy of The Very Little Theatre.*

A cloche hat, as featured in a 1925 issue of *Ladies' Home Journal.*

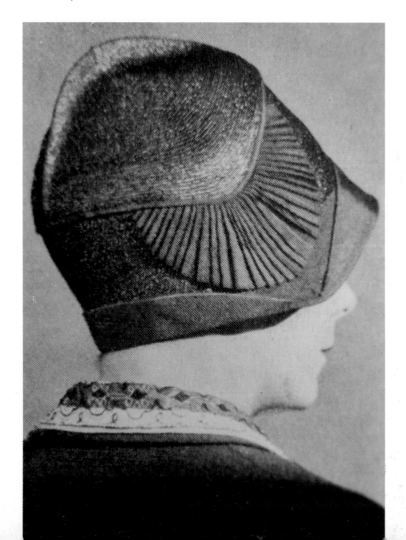

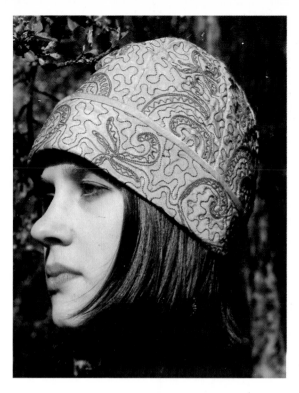

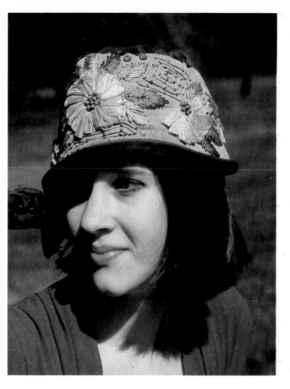

This cloche has such a full brim that it was probably originally worn by a woman who refused to bob her hair. *Courtesy of The Very Little Theatre.*

With nearly every type of needlework trim imaginable (including beading, embroidery, and appliqué), this cloche is a testament to one needlewoman's skill. *Courtesy of The Very Little Theatre.*

A straw cloche trimmed with fat feathers, from *Ladies' Home Journal.*

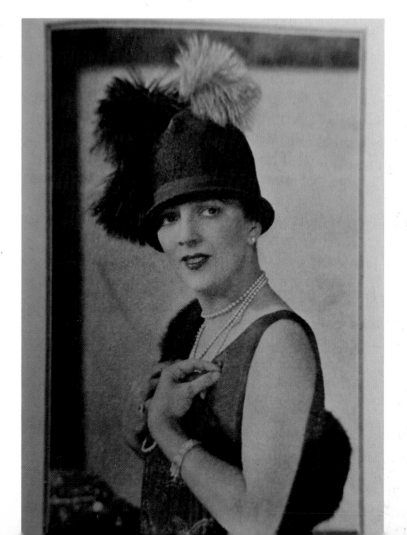

A gold metallic cloche. *Courtesy of The Very Little Theatre.*

A black velvet and satin cloche garnished with embroidery. *Courtesy of The Very Little Theatre.*

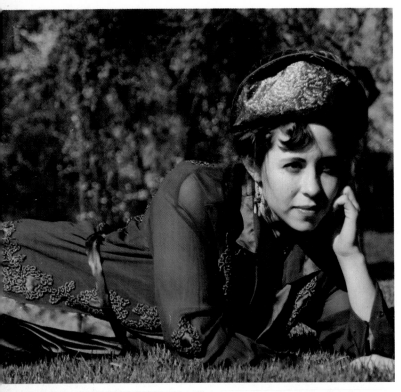

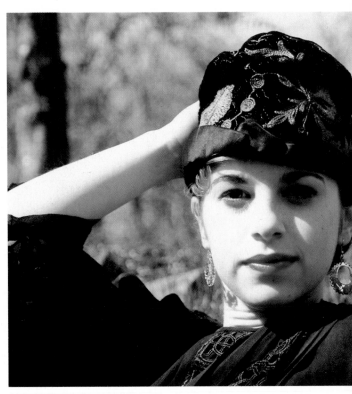

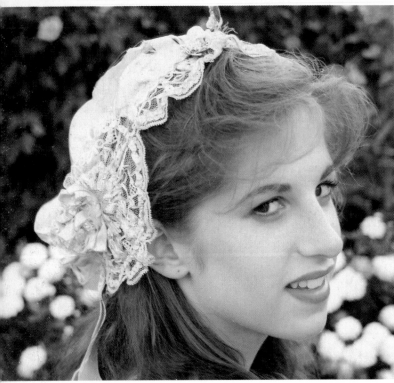

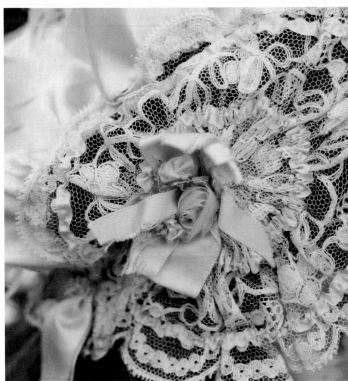

A boudoir cap of silk, trimmed with detailed lace and ribbon rosettes. *Courtesy of The Very Little Theatre.*

A circa 1921 brimmed hat of satin and brocade. *Courtesy of The Very Little Theatre.*

A soft, brimmed hat from the early twenties. *Courtesy of The Very Little Theatre.*

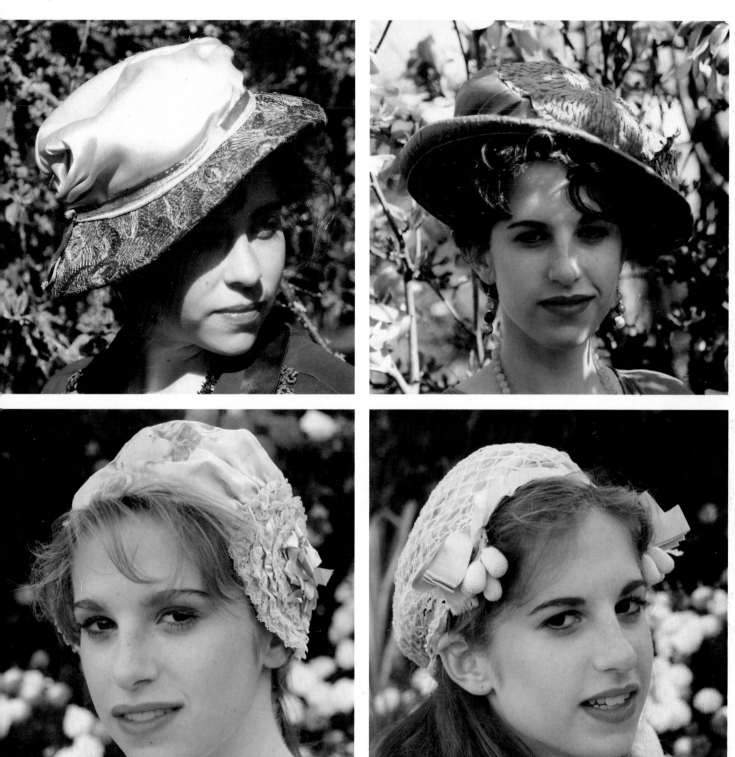

A printed silk boudoir cap embellished with lace and ribbon trim. *Courtesy of The Very Little Theatre.*

A home-made boudoir cap crocheted over baby blue silk. *Courtesy of The Very Little Theatre.*

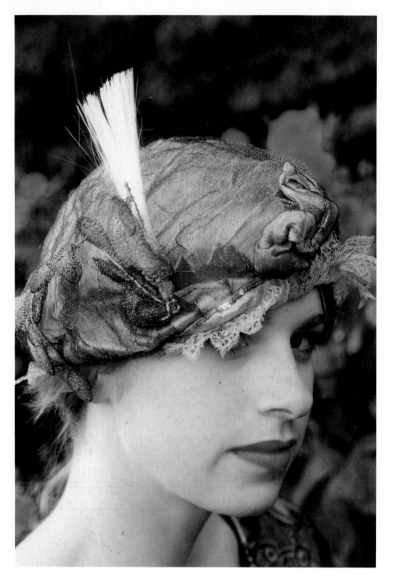

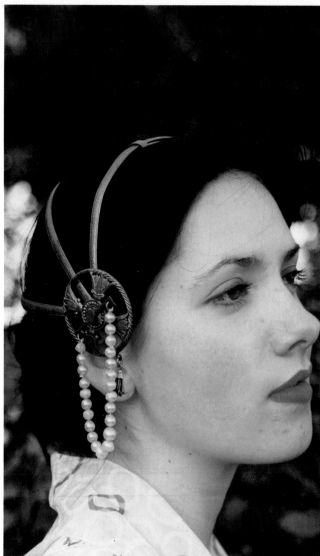

An evening cap circa 1919–1920. Made of gold satin and metallic-shot lace, the cap features a metal wire and bristle bird. *Courtesy of The Very Little Theatre.*

A metal headpiece dripping with faux pearls and Egyptian-inspired motifs. *Courtesy of Persona Vintage Clothing.*

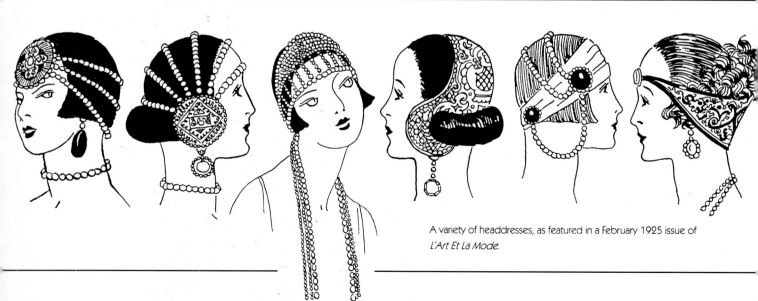

A variety of headdresses, as featured in a February 1925 issue of *L'Art Et La Mode.*

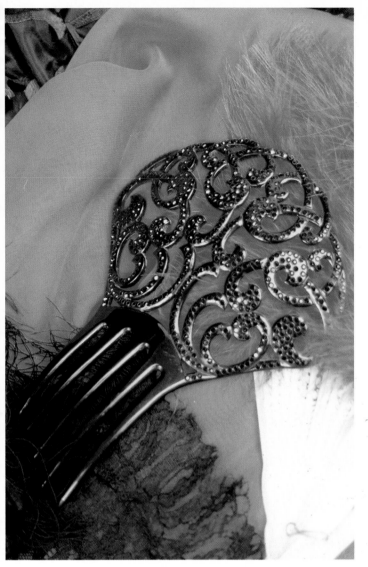
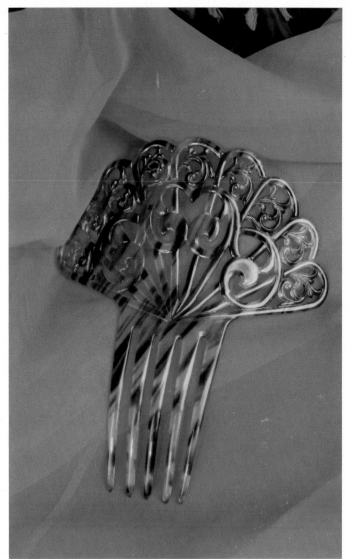

Celluloid hair combs, measuring approximately eight inches in length. Worn high on the head, they looked like regal crowns.

Evening fans, from *L'Art Et La Mode*.

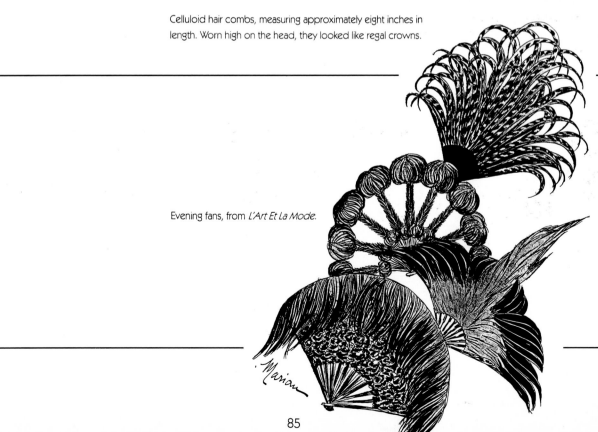

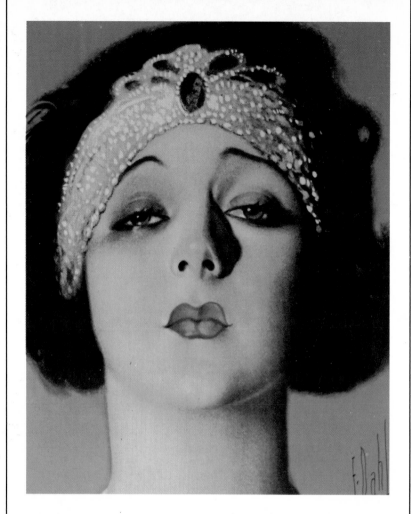

A rhinestone and paste-jewel headdress from 1925, as featured
on the cover of *Motion Picture Classic*.

Following Page:
A scarf headdress, as featured on a song sheet from the era.

A turban-style headdress.

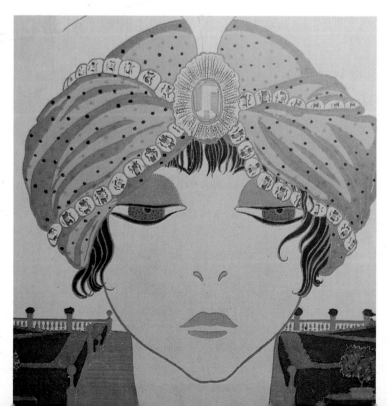

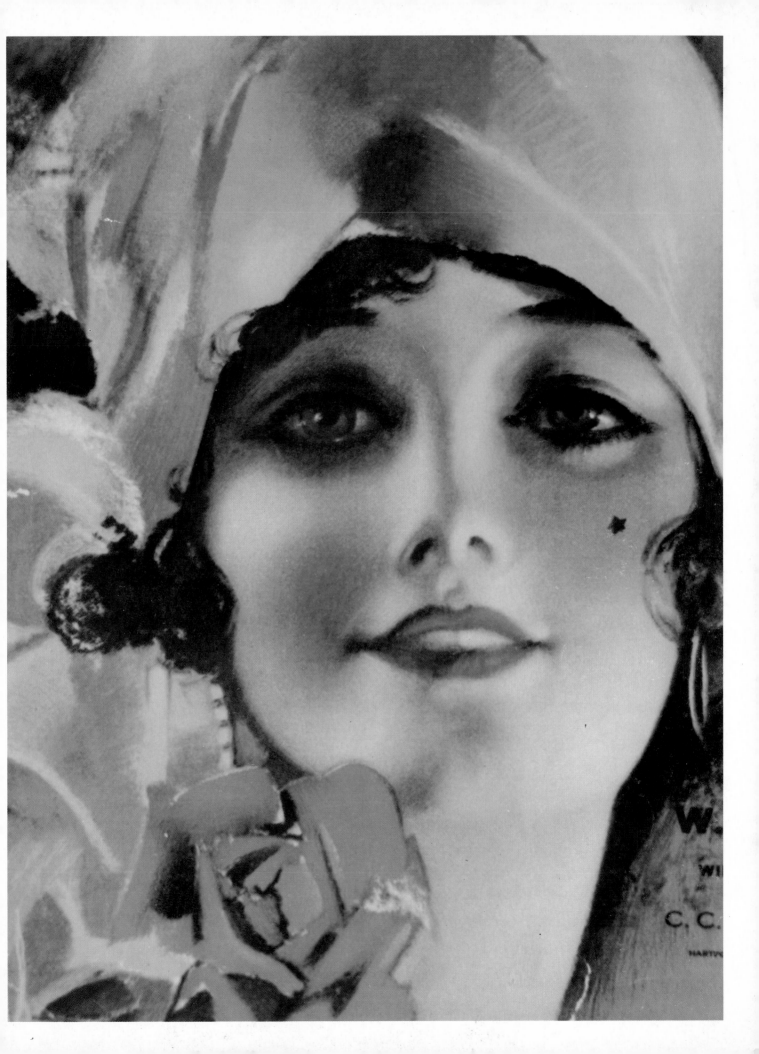

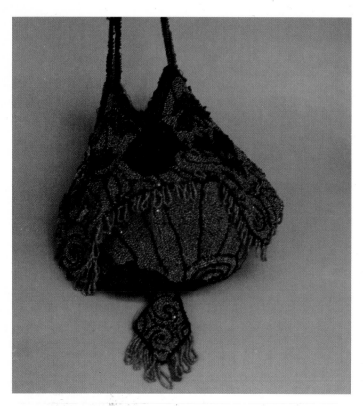

A circa 1920 beaded reticule bag. *Courtesy of The Very Little Theatre.*

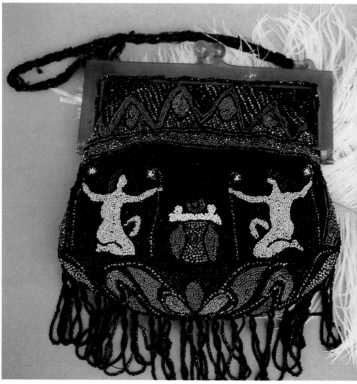

A beaded bag with a celluloid clasp showing strong influence from ancient Egypt. *Courtesy of The Very Little Theatre.*

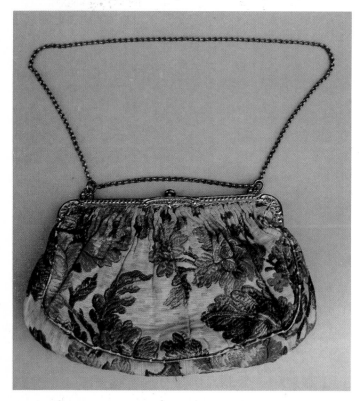

A brocade bag with a metal clasp and shoulder chain. *Courtesy of The Very Little Theatre.*

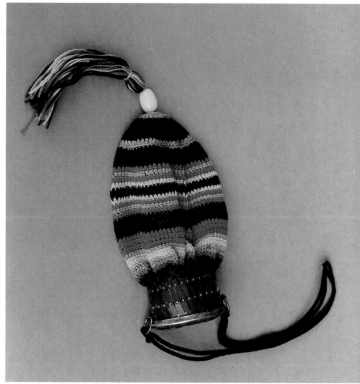

Above and Right: Though the metal closure on this bag features an Art Nouveau (turn-of-the-century) design, the style and colors of the body of the bag are more characteristic of the 1920s. Quite possibly, the frame of the bag was recycled in the 1920s. *Courtesy of The Very Little Theatre.*

An early twenties reticule purse of painted silk with clear beading embellishment. *Courtesy of The Very Little Theatre.*

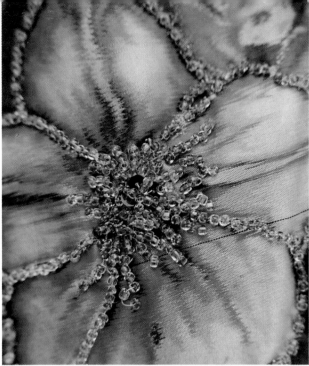

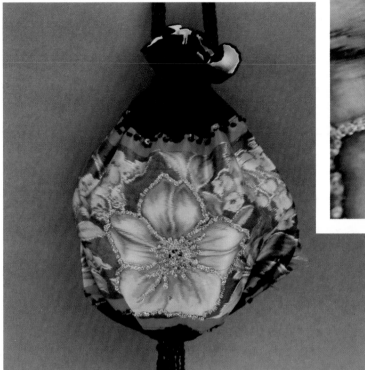

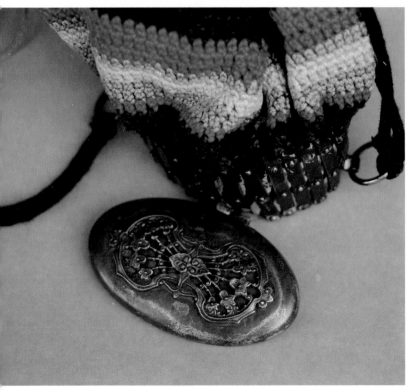

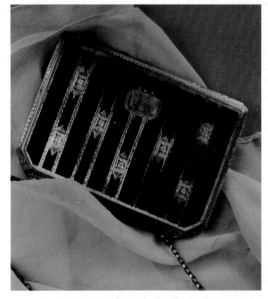

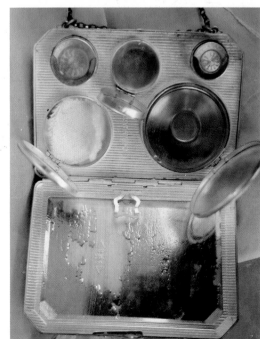

Above right and Right: A circa 1920 metal handbag. When opened, this handy accessory features a mirror (foil-backed and now partially peeled away), a bill clip, two change holders, and three make-up holders (probably for powder, rouge, and lip color). *Courtesy of The Very Little Theatre.*

89

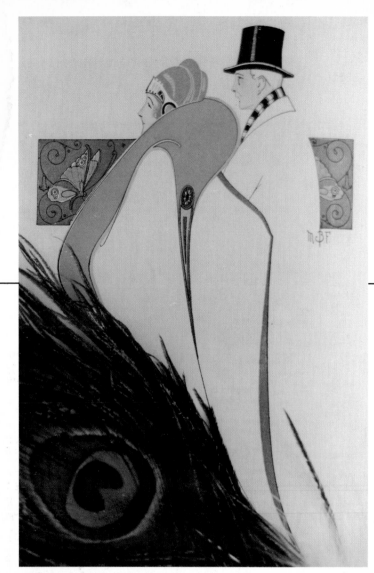

Evening capes were often large, full, and sophisticated. This one was featured in a 1925 advertisement for Colgate's Perfumes.

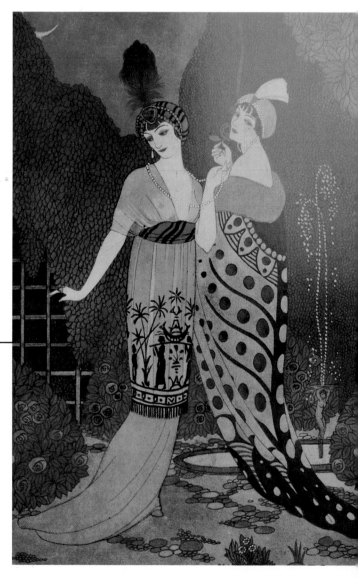

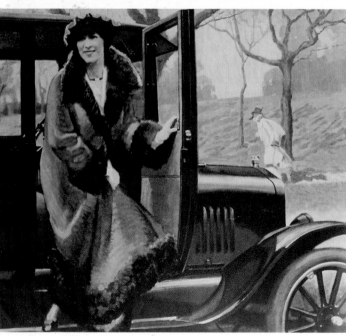

As seen in a 1925 advertisement for the Ford Car Company, "everyday" coats were often heavy and trimmed with fur.

Though draped and wrapped cocoon coats (like the one shown on the right) were most favored in the late 'teens, women still clung to them early in the twenties.

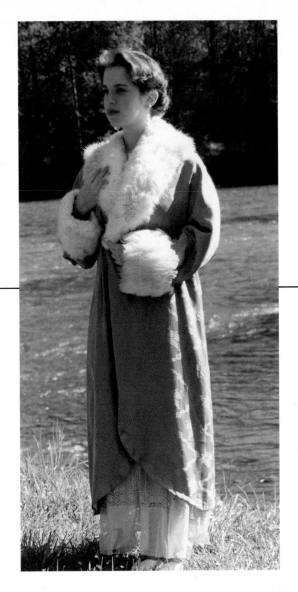

A satin coat trimmed with fur. *Courtesy of The Very Little Theatre.*

This full, deeply fringed cape dates to circa 1920. *Courtesy of The Very Little Theatre.*

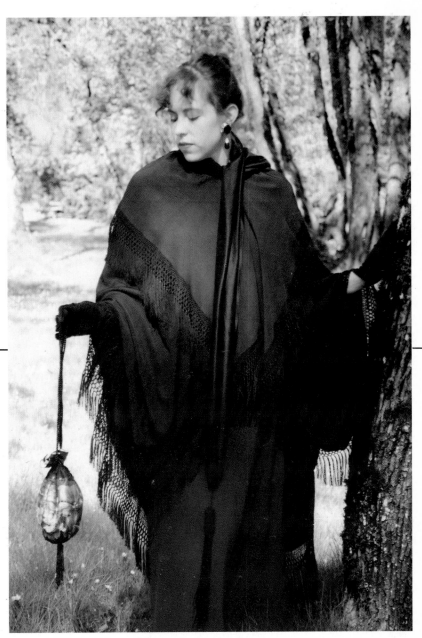

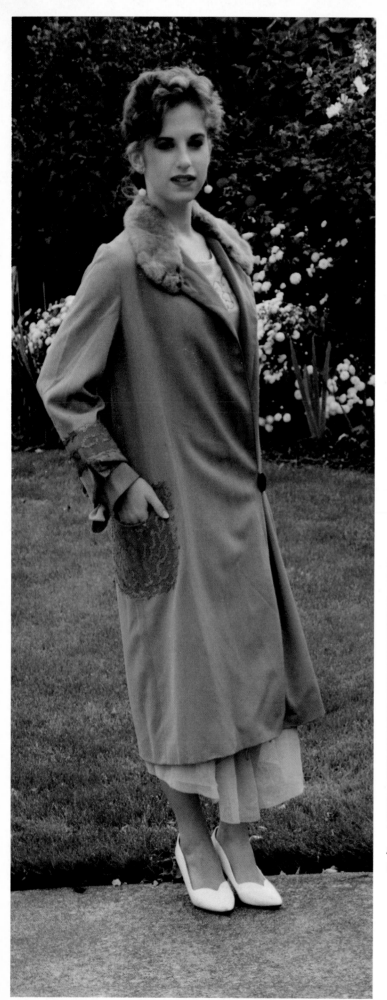

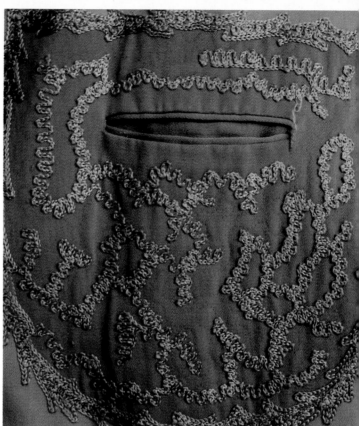

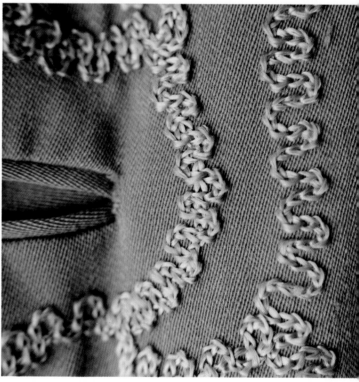

An unusually detailed coat embellished with braid and appliqué.
Courtesy of The Very Little Theatre.

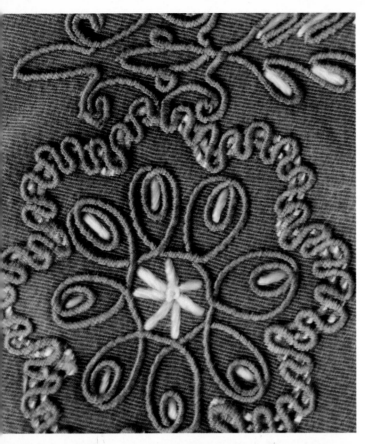

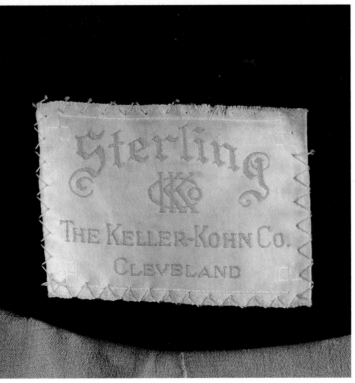

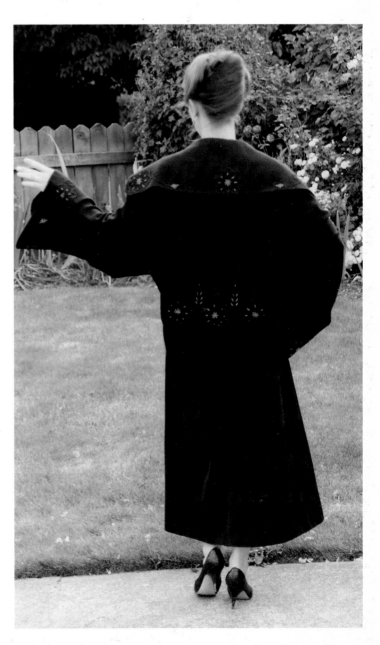

An elegant garment which must have been posh in its time. A great deal of braid and cord work embellishes the coat. *Courtesy of The Very Little Theatre.*

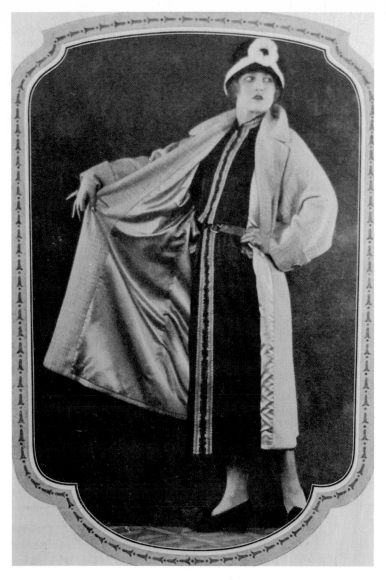

A simple coat with a rich satin lining, as featured in a Skinner's Satins advertisement.

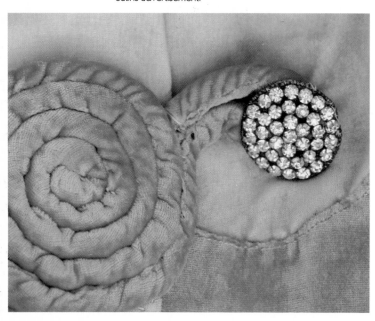

A plush velour coat in shades of orange. The clasps are creative and unusual. *Courtesy of The Very Little Theatre.*

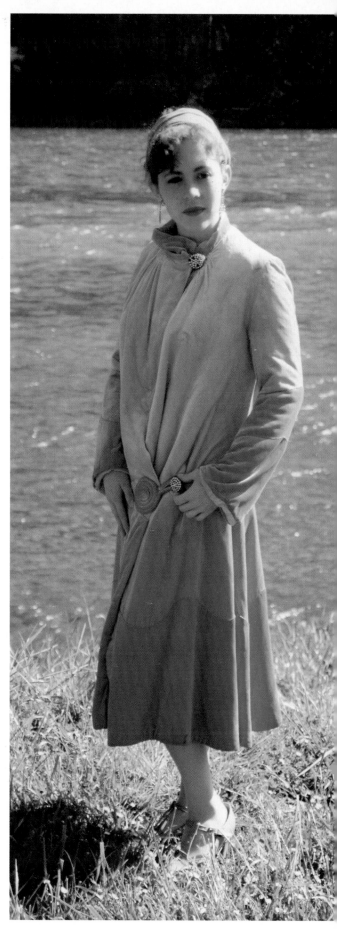

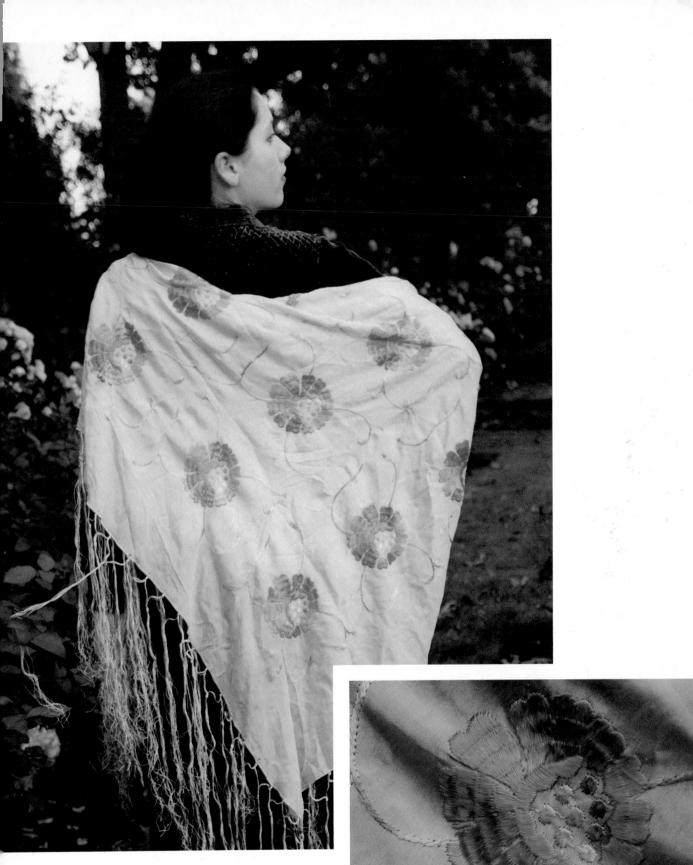

A silk shawl with a machine-embroidered design. *Courtesy of The Very Little Theatre.*

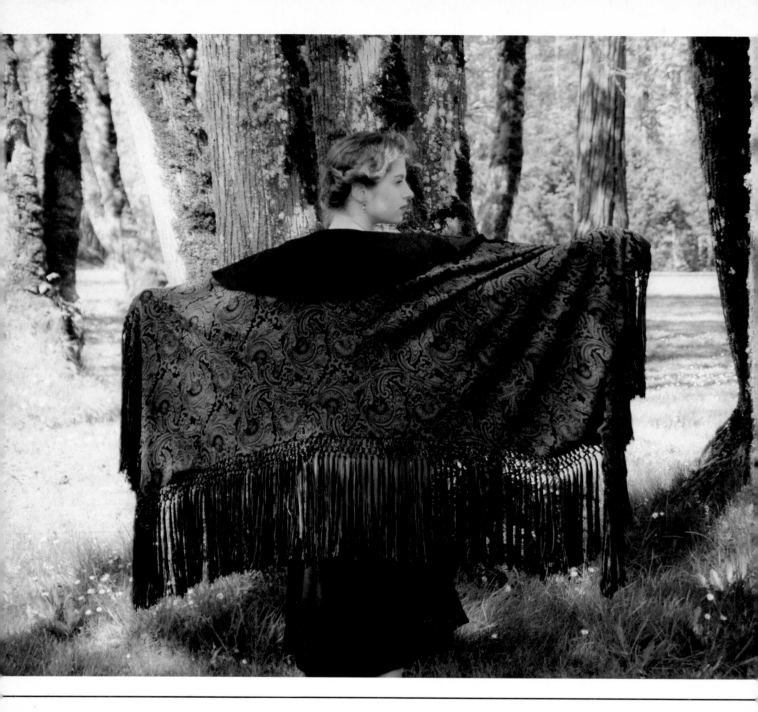

An exquisite wool paisley shawl with deep fringe. *Courtesy of The Very Little Theatre.*

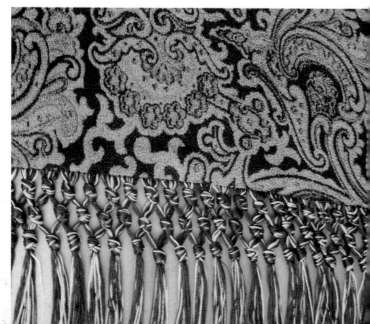

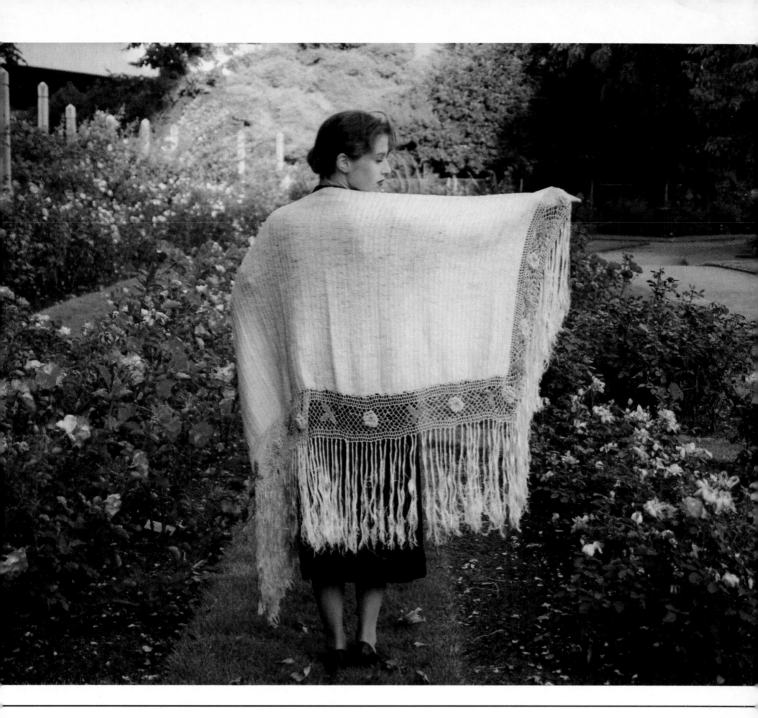

A home-made shawl of fine wool and cashmere. *Courtesy of The Very Little Theatre.*

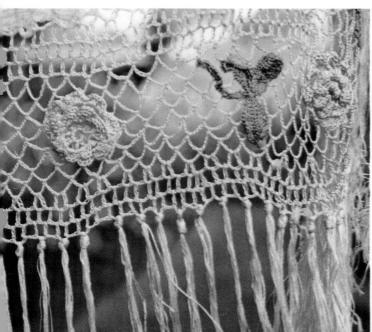

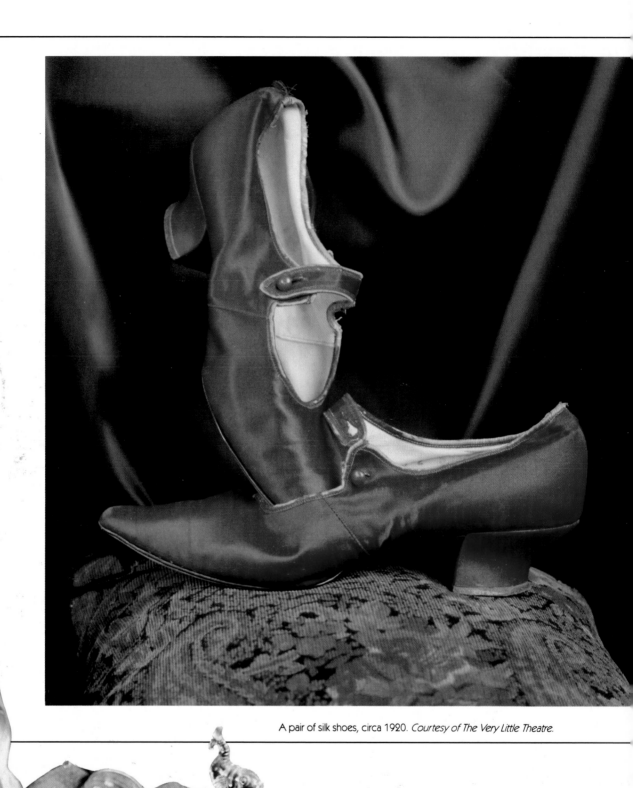

A pair of silk shoes, circa 1920. *Courtesy of The Very Little Theatre.*

Gold brocade shoes from late in the decade. *Courtesy of The Very Little Theatre.*

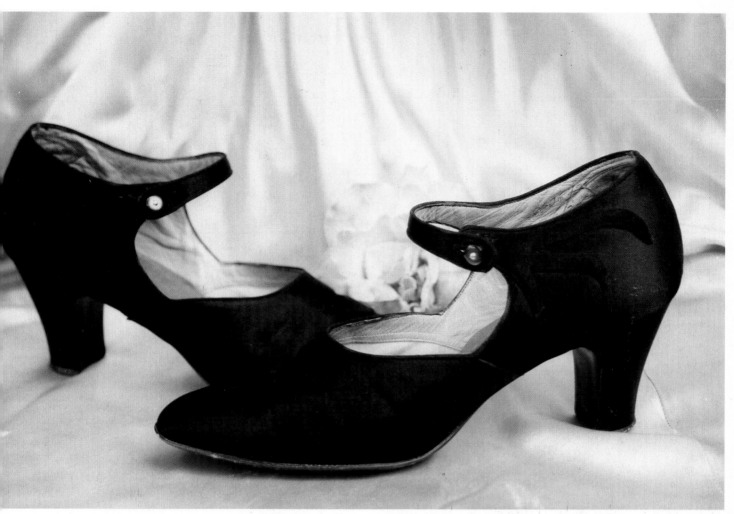

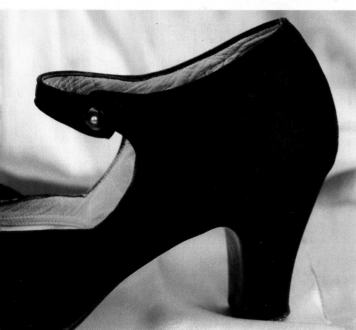

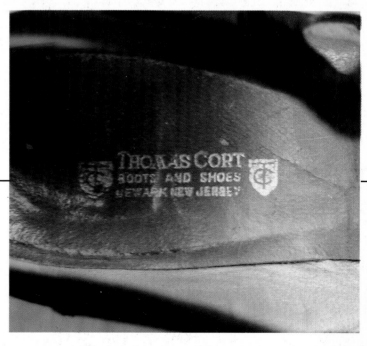

Satin shoes with a "wave" of Art Deco flair.

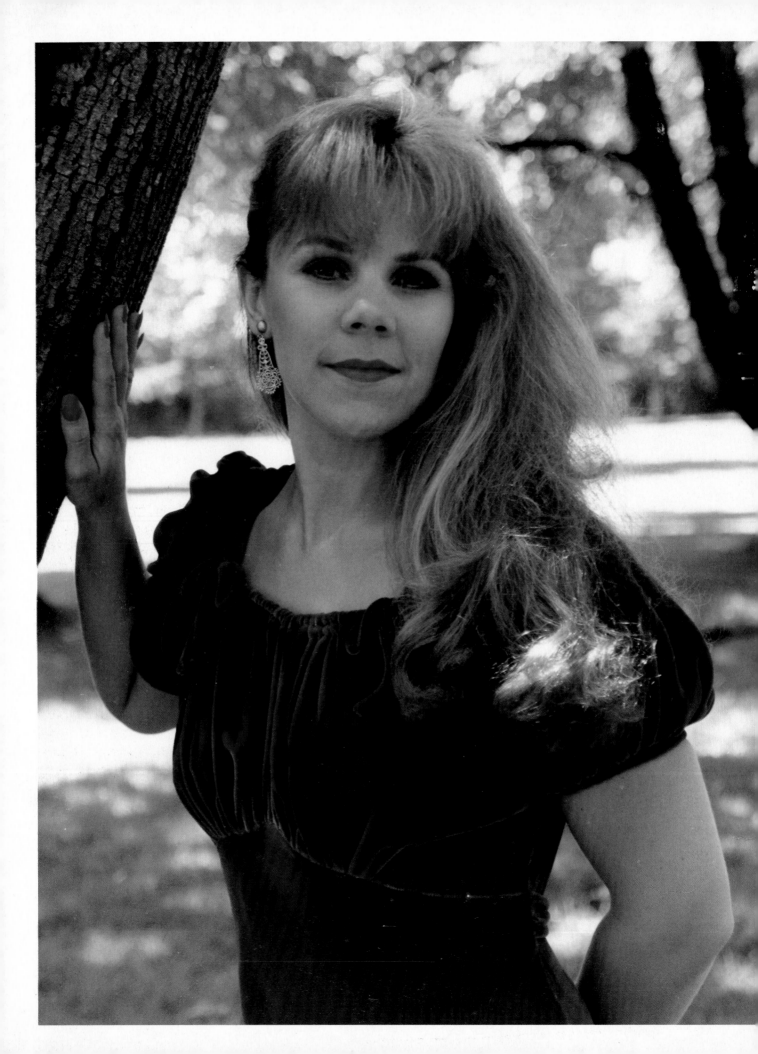

CHAPTER FIVE

1930S: GLAMOUR GIRL

"Glamour is all!" *Vogue* proclaimed in 1935. Red lips and nails were now part of nearly every woman's dress, and for the first time fashion magazines were describing clothing as "sexy." "Sex appeal is the prime motif," *Vogue* elaborated later in the decade, "and sex appeal is no longer a matter of subtle appeal." Women were women again. Finally tired of speaking of "lines" and "angles," the woman of the thirties made certain her every curve was not only seen, but emphasized; the new fashions were cut to fit smoothly over a rounded bustline and curving hips.

"A woman can never be too rich or too thin" became the motto of the decade. Dieting—and fasting—became the new past–time for fashionable women. In keeping with a song that insisted women must "keep young and beautiful if you want to be loved," a fitness craze swept over America and Europe. "Your very important profile will have the windswept, fleet lines of a speedboat or aeroplane," British *Vogue* decreed in 1934. Like all else in this increasingly technical decade, in order to be modern, women had to be "streamlined."

But despite fashion magazine's glamour and glitz, the 1930s was a troubled era in American history, beginning with the Great Depression and ending with the start of World War II. Movie houses hosted films featuring heavily made–up, seductive actresses like Greta Garbo, Tallulah Bankhead, Mae West, and Jean Harlow. The characters they portrayed wore glittering costumes and lived in fairy-tale–like stories, in which money problems were soon (and miraculously) resolved; their clothes and their lives were very *unlike* those of the average woman.

Even the woman who could afford gorgeous designer fashions had to deal with a society that frowned upon such designs, because the new fashions were seen as either too extravagant or decidedly "naughty." Queen Mary believed the latter, and soon banned low-backed and -fronted dresses from her court. She also warned court attendants that make-up disturbed her.

"These are not ordinary times," Sears catalog conceded in their 1932 catalog, "We realize that economy dictates that women must sew more this year . . . Repairing, rather than replacing, will be the order in many families." Ironically, though, garments of the thirties required *more* fabric than fashions of the previous decade. Still, while the new look may have been much more feminine, and perhaps even less economical, it was definitely a more sober, adult look. Thicker fabrics and a new innovation—the shoulder pad—helped women bear the burden of the increasingly difficult world around them.

DRESSES

For perhaps the first time in history, the thirties brought about a marked difference between what women wore by day and what they wore in the evening. Simple, practical, somewhat dowdy dresses were the fashion of daytime, but at night, glamour and fantasy ruled. Even the working girl could afford one simple yet elegant evening gown, in slinky, shiny black satin.

Even so, financial hardship shows on most of the fashions that exist from the period. Chemise dresses from the twenties are found with middles altered to indent at the waist, and layers of ruffles added at the hem and sleeves. Sewing books from the period are heavily centered on revamping and restyling old clothes. Hand-me-downs were very close to being fashionable. As home-sewing reached new levels of popularity, Sears catalog even featured "semi-made" garments that could be purchased less expensively than ready-to-wear, but still saved sewers time. Already cut out, and with more difficult areas (including those with tucking, pleating, or tailoring) already sewn, all that was necessary was to sew up the side seams, sleeves, and hem. Sears claimed the system saved their buyers "at least 1/3" the cost of a ready-made garment.

For those who could not sew, the ready-made market was increasingly a source for every type of garment—and the best ready-mades were sewn so well it became increasingly difficult to distinguish them from a house-designer model. Although ready-to-wear was growing in popularity, it had many hurdles yet to jump. In the twenties, sizing had been easy; small, medium, and large was all that was needed for non–fitted che-

Previous page:
Velvet evening gowns from the 1930s are plentiful today. *Courtesy of The Very Little Theatre.*

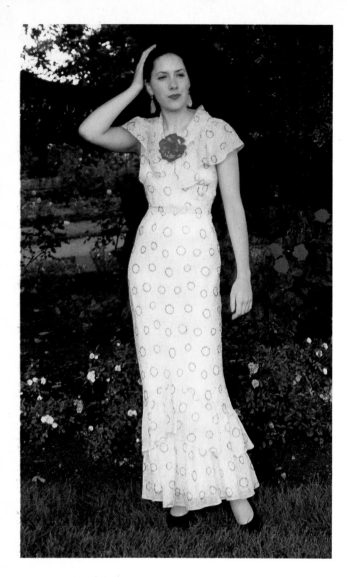

Spanish influence shines through in this vivid dress. *Courtesy of Persona Vintage Clothing.*

mise dresses. In the thirties, when dresses were designed to fit smoothly on the figure, sizing was only a tad more accurate—and department stores made good use of their alterations departments. Smallish shoulder pads (an innovation credited to designer Schiaparelli, but whose origin is obscure) designed to softly round the shoulder-line, made this fitting a little easier; by diminishing or enlarging the shoulder pad, the fit of the shoulders, arm cycle, and bustline could all be affected.

"ZIP...open! ZIP...closed! That's the smart, smooth, modern way!" one 1930 ad raved about the effectiveness of the zipper. Still, while the so-called "hookless fastener" had been invented in the 1890s, by the 1930s it was still being used only in accessories—until Schiaparelli incorporated it into her line of couture clothing. By the end of the decade, ready-to-wear garments often featured zippers and most women agreed with fashion illustrator Marcel Vertes: "That little diabolic 'Sesame' that shuts you in or out" was grand!

Another innovation of the 1930s also had its origin in an earlier decade. The bias-cut, for all intents and purposes, was invented around 1919, but it wasn't until the thirties that it was used to good advantage and became all-important to the fashionable look. Actually, many dresses of the thirties differ little from chemise dresses of the twenties; in fact, when examined off of a human figure, dresses of the early thirties are easily mistaken for those of the 1920s. It was only the bias-cut, as introduced by Madame Vionnet, that made those tube-dresses *cling* when worn.

Another subtle detail that made thirties dresses different was the re-introduction of the waistline. In the first few years of the decade, this was almost exclusively seen as an upside-down triangle that clung to the waist and pointed to the hem. Later, around 1934, the triangle was reversed, pointing to the face. By 1936 fashion magazines were talking about "indented waists," and by 1939 a new, wasp-waisted, squared-shoulder look was beginning to take hold—until World War II ended any influence of impractical nipped-waist designs.

Shirtwaist dresses made their first all-practical appearance in the thirties, and were originally called "Louisa May Alcott day dresses." In response to the new need for practical, lasting styles, quilted dresses were briefly revived.

In the evening, formal dresses turned old-fashioned and long—sometimes even with Victorian-style trains. Halter necklines appeared, as did backless designs (making it tempting to enter the room backwards!). Beaded dresses continued in their popularity, and although there was now more dress to bead, beaded gowns could usually be purchased less expensively than they had been in the twenties. For the most part, this was because manufacturers had discovered less labor-intensive, time–consuming methods. Rarely were dresses hand-beaded anymore—machines did most of the work. Similarly, so-called "dance dresses" were inexpensively made by machine in the "fish scale" look. This all-over style of applying sequins made the dresses extremely heavy, but they were particularly popular. "Sequins flash like a glance from a bright eye, and kill their man at ten yards—" *Vogue* raved.

As technology made leaps and bounds forward, synthetic fabrics became the heroes of hard economic times; less expensive and easy to care for, rayons and acetates abounded. One new, particularly popular fabric was "laquered satin." It was available mostly in black, and was somewhat stiff and extremely shiny—making it ideal for the ever-popular slinky black evening gown. Still, good old cottons, linens, and wools were used extensively because of their longevity—even by couture designers. Muted colors, particularly in black, navy, grey, and shades of brown were favorites for "everyday" clothes.

Skirts & Slacks

By 1929, hemlines crashed to the floor, to be worn calf–length by day, floor length by night. Those who could not afford the new, longer styles added ruffles and flounces to their tubular 1920s skirts, but even couture fashion magazines featured brand new skirts suffocated with flounces. Gone was the shapeless tube of a skirt. The new style hugged the hips, bowed slightly along the thigh, and burst open just below the knee.

Later in the decade, as the Depression persisted, all flounces and fluff were removed from the skirt, making it long, curving, and streamlined. And there skirts stayed for most of the decade, until around 1939 when skirts rose a full fifteen to seventeen inches from the floor.

Offering some competition to the skirt, slacks began to emerge as more than just sportswear. Though still reserved for the casual moments in life, figure–flattering slacks that fit smoothly over the hips and gracefully plummeted to the ankles in a full bell–bottom style were readily adopted by most women for playful outings.

By 1930, Sears could see the future of slacks for women: "Overalls for women!" the catalog headline read. "Dainty, fadeproof colors . . . Everybody's wearing them! They're all the rage . . .The most exclusive shops on Fifth Avenue are selling them! . . . At the beach—in the garden or laundry—at house-cleaning—for camping and touring—in stores—industrial work . . . Rose, Orchid, Tan, Blue, Green or Peach."

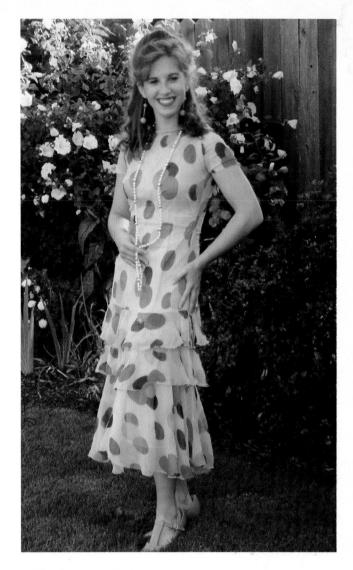

A chiffon dress trimmed with flounces, circa 1929–1930. *Courtesy of The Very Little Theatre.*

Blouses

Moderate necklines that (in day wear at least) rarely scooped farther than the collar bone, wider shoulders, bows tied and drooping at the base of the neck, sailor collars, Peter Pan collars, softly pointed collars . . . all drew the onlooker's eye *above* the waistline. By evening, novel sleeves trimmed with scallops, ruching, or puffs pulled the same trick, as did draped or cowl necklines. Arguably, the blouse had become the most important part of women's dress.

For "dressy" occasions, a new innovation—dress clips—added further detail to the blouse. Made of paste rhinestones and faux pearls, these innovative pieces of jewelry literally clipped onto either side of a scooping or sweetheart neckline—a style that would persist into the next decade.

Shoulders grew increasingly broad during the decade, and by 1934, most detail on blouses was designed to emphasize this feature. (Even the revers on women's jackets were designed to point up to the shoulder, not down to the waist as they had previously.)

Though the style of knitted garments such as sweaters, berets, undergarments, and gloves had been popular since the 'teens, knitted garments took on new importance during the 1930s, as homemade styles became essential for many women. Even *Vogue* acknowledged this trend. "Sweaters appear, tough as you please, forever and a day, with our tweed skirts, with our golfing slacks. They appear, in highly sophisticated versions, with our town suits," the editors commented in 1939. "Their social climb touches its peak when they appear, loaded with jewels, slashed with silk, over a grandly outsized evening skirt."

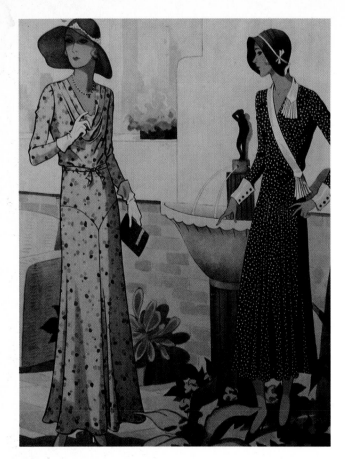

Day dresses like these are difficult for collectors to find today, due to the economic pressures of the era; most often, they were worn until they fell apart—or, they were never created because old clothes had to "make do." Notice that tiny prints prevail, and pointed, low waistlines are featured in this McCall Pattern Company sewing pattern plate.

Lingerie

"You must not let a little thing like a wasp–waist frighten you in the least," British *Vogue* insisted in 1939. "And don't let anyone picture a modern woman gasping for breath. Nowadays clever corsets ease you gently into the silhouette that used to be achieved with a coat of armor." Though it was true that the new corsets were a far cry from their heavily boned Victorian ancestors, one could hardly call the waist of the 1930s "waspish." Early in the decade, a very natural (sometimes rather wide) waist was favored. Girdle–like corsets, very much like those worn in the 1920s, did little more than gently smooth the silhouette.

Little by little, however, the waist did whittle itself into a slightly more indented feature, with the help of featherboning stitched into corsets along the sides of the waist. Late in 1939 true, heavily boned, laced-up, Victorian-style corsets did appear—but were quickly abandoned when war broke out.

The newest innovation in corsets was the zipper; and while women would later wonder what they ever did without the little contraption, saleswomen in the 1930s were instructed to teach women how to operate the unfamiliar gadget.

Other undergarments stayed largely the same in the 1930s as they had been in the 1920s, though they had a tendency to be less elaborate—void of embroideries and frills. Still, with new emphasis being placed on the bustline, slips adopted wider bust darts for definition. Likewise, with the waist now emerging, waistlines on slips often had a pointed and gently fitted middle.

And then there was the bra. A teenager named Mary Jacob invented the modern bra when her corset cover seemed conspicuous under a peek-a-boo dress; succinctly she pinned two handkerchiefs together and tied them around her body. Later she said "the result was delicious. I could move more freely, a nearly naked feeling." She patented the design in 1913, but it wasn't until the 1930s, when curves became important for the first time in some twenty years, that bras finally appeared as a staple of women's wear. Cup sizes were created. The "uplift" bra made its first appearance. And circular stitching (usually associated with bras of the late 1940s and 1950s) appeared.

Leisure Wear

"In 1931 [the] 'dinner pajama' made its bid for a place in the limelight," author Carrie Hall recalled in her book of fashion reminiscences. This new-style, elegant housedress "was a long, bifurcated underslip with a long coatlike robe of chiffon, fluffily trimmed. The 1933 interpretation...was called a house coat or hostess gown. These evolved into the tea dinner gown of 1936, which, because of its smartness, it becomingness, and its convenience—it could be worn for dinner at home—was considered the last word in swanky attire."

The dinner pajama and its successors were not the only advances made in casual wear, however. While pants were frequently worn for extremely casual affairs, a new type of dress dubbed the "sundress" appeared for casual occasions when women still wanted to look pretty and feminine.

After great strides in sportswear in the 1920s, there was little left for the woman of the thirties to want for when she golfed, skated, or (as was the trend) played tennis. But bathing suit manufactures outdid themselves. Extinct were the bloomers or leggings that had concealed female bather's legs for over six decades. Dead and buried were any trace of sleeves. Necklines scooped dangerously low on many suits, and backs often disappeared altogether. Though more simple than ever, bathing suits revealed more than any man had ever hoped to glimpse on a public beach.

By the early thirties, Jantzen had a firm hold on the swim-suit industry, and their suits were considered the best available. Many of their designs were on the cutting edge, and their fabrics and quality were superior. Jantzen appears to have been the first swimsuit manufacturer to use "Lastex" and "Contralex" in their suits—which women loved, since these helped slim down their figures the way a girdle did.

In 1935, the bikini appeared—and though it was worn only by a few daring women because it was considered very revealing, leaving "some inches of flesh exposed between its two parts," it was modest by today's standards. As the "revealing" look in swimwear became increasingly "shocking," Jantzen introduced a new, revolutionary bathing suit called the "wisp-o-weight." Designed to show as much flesh as was legally possible, the "wisp-o-weight" had added appeal: it was available in flesh tones (among other modern colors), so the bathing beauty who donned it appeared—at first glance, at least—to be nude.

Soon enough, however, the women of the thirties had as much flesh in the sun and sand as they could stand, and by 1938, bathing suits were most fashionable if they had some feminine touches—including short skirts.

OTHER IMPORTANT GARMENTS

As manufacturers became increasingly engrossed in creating man-made fabrics, a myriad of new materials became available. A few became staples, but many never fully caught on despite big promotional ad campaigns. One new man-made material that did have a lasting affect, however, was a specially manufactured cellophane, first introduced as "Rhodophane." This was, in fact, the first see-through plastic-like fabric, and was soon all the rage for rain hoods, capes, and umbrellas.

Even more notably, at the 1939 New York World's Fair, nylon stockings were introduced. Clinging to the leg as well as (or perhaps better than) silk stockings, the "nylons" were an instant hit, and over 64 million pairs—marketed as "run-resistant"—were sold.

Shoes from the 1930s are very similar to those from the 1920s, though more sleek styles—often without straps—predominated. Open-toed and platform shoes also appeared in the late 1930s, and by 1939 *Vogue* proclaimed that "nothing is dowdier than a dainty foot."

Hats were by far the most intriguing accessory available: Everything from "Princess Eugenie" hats (little round hats with tiny brims and loads of feathers), to berets, pillboxes, tricorns, "Scarlett O'Hara" wide-brims, and what British *Vogue* described as "giant flat phonograph discs" worn tilted to one side of the head. The more unique, fun, and striking, the more the hat was favored.

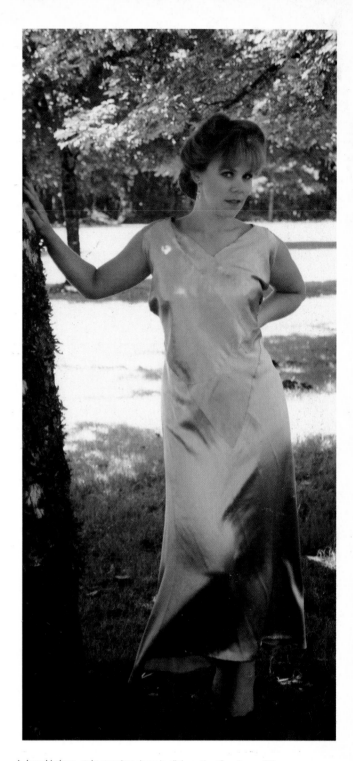

A Jean Harlow–style evening dress in slinky satin. *Courtesy of The Very Little Theatre.*

To compliment the mode for hats, women wore gloves when wishing to look particularly chic. Worn in shades to match shoes, many day gloves were made of cotton, or knitted at home, while gloves worn in the evening where usually long and made up in satins or other lush fabrics.

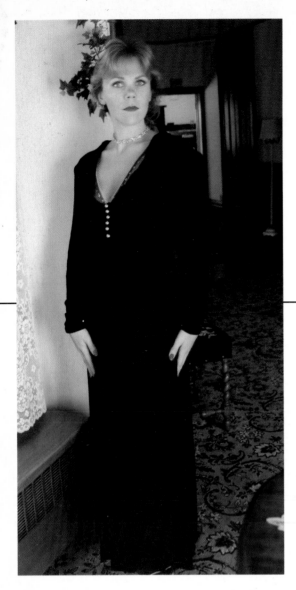

A rich, elegant velvet dress with a gold metallic shot bodice worn under a matching velvet bolero. *Courtesy of The Very Little Theatre.*

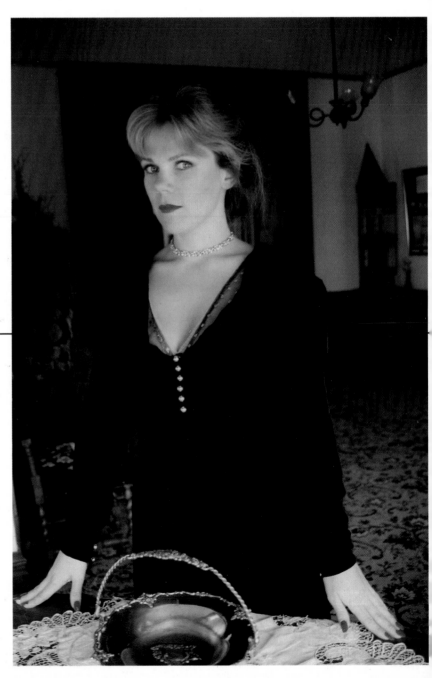

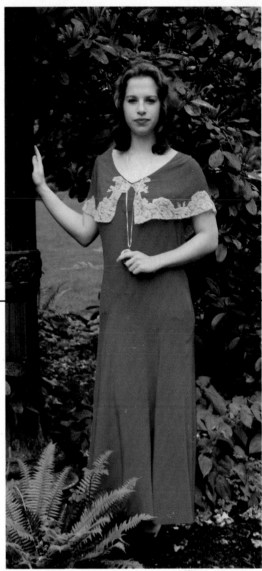

A brilliantly shaded rayon dress with a shaped waist and wide collar, circa 1930. *Courtesy of The Very Little Theatre.*

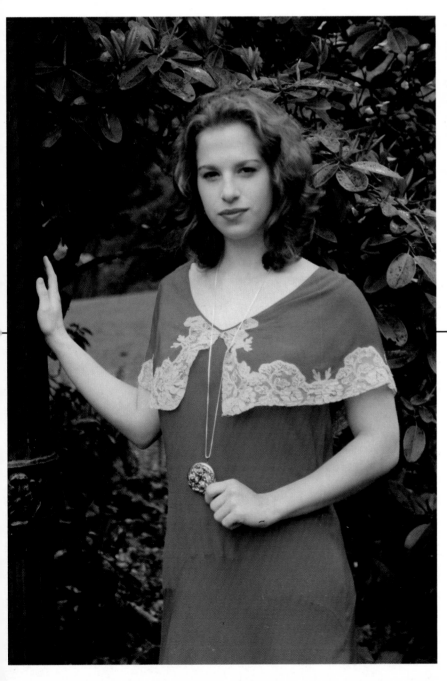

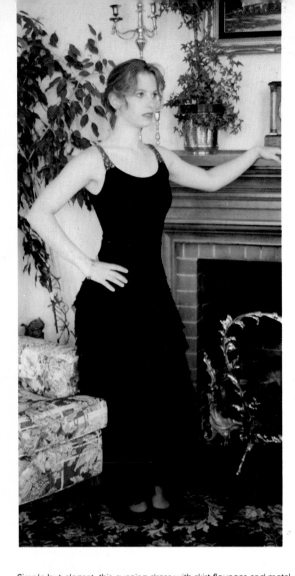

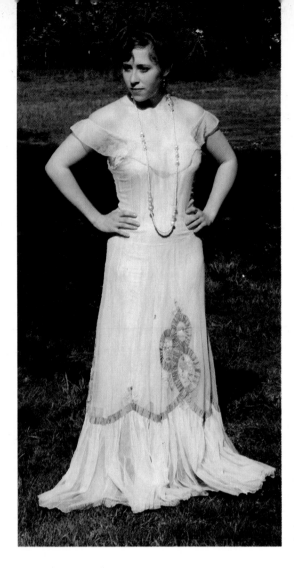

Simple but elegant, this evening dress with skirt flounces and metal beading at the shoulder straps dates to circa 1930. *Courtesy of Persona Vintage Clothing.*

Femininity was revived in the 1930s with neo-Victorian styles. This dress is of fine ecru netting and is embellished with ribbon trim and embroidery. *Courtesy of The Very Little Theatre.*

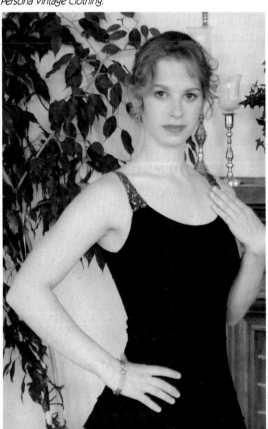

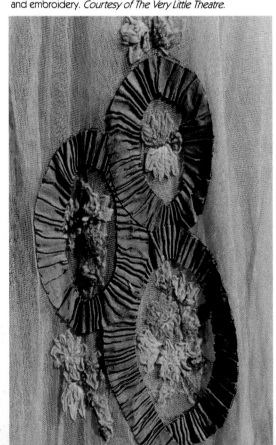

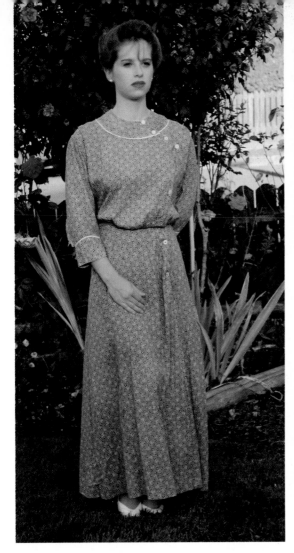

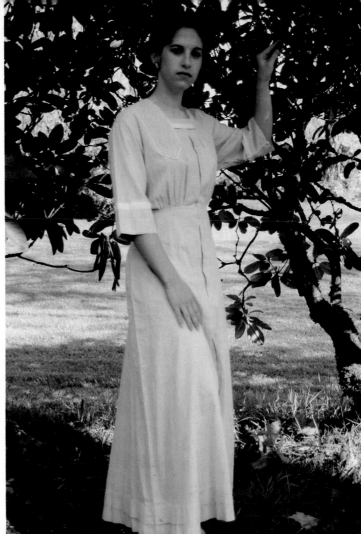

Many women wore dresses like these everyday. Though they bear little resemblance to fashion plates of the period, they were sturdy and practical. *Courtesy of The Very Little Theatre.*

Daywear featured in the McCall Pattern Company catalog.

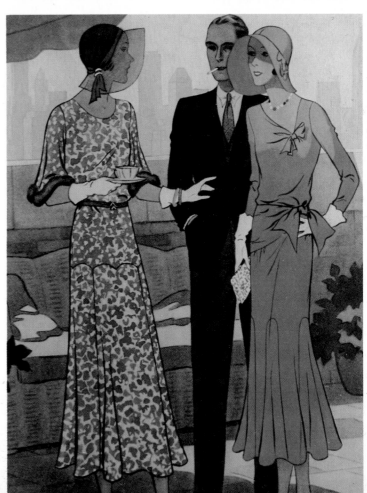

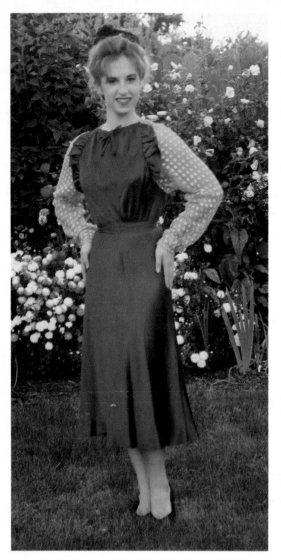
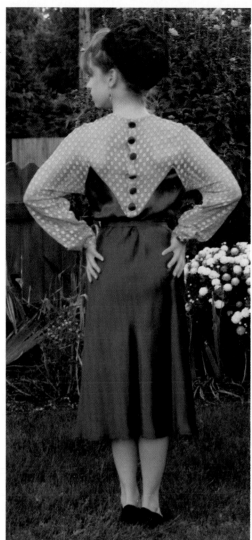
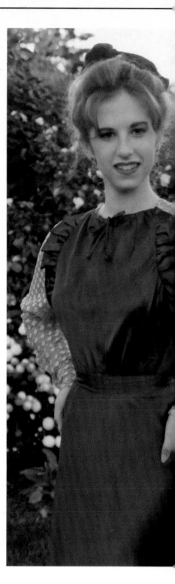

Many unusual and unique dress styles can be found in 1930s evening wear. This one is of satin and net. Courtesy of The Very Little Theatre.

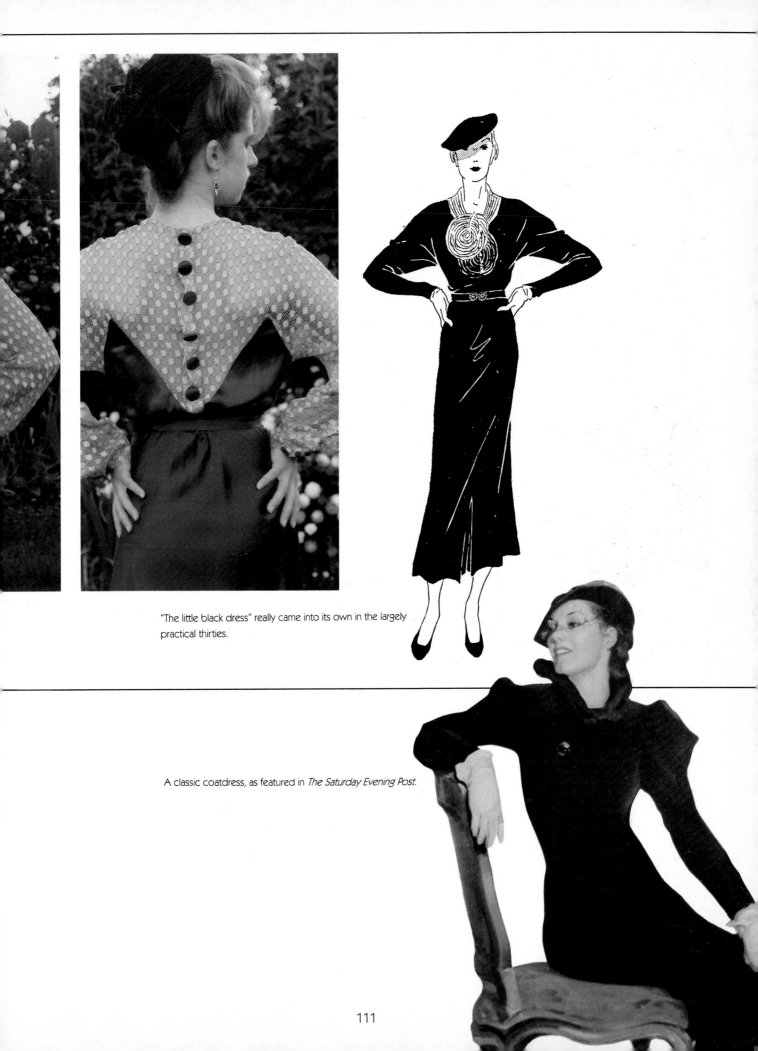

"The little black dress" really came into its own in the largely practical thirties.

A classic coatdress, as featured in *The Saturday Evening Post*.

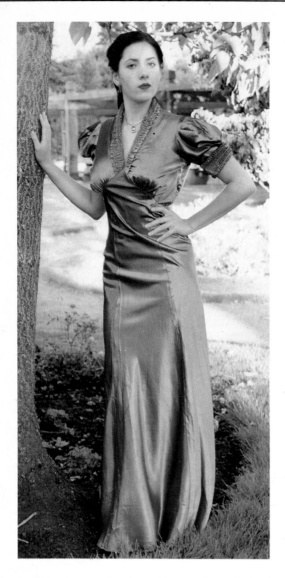

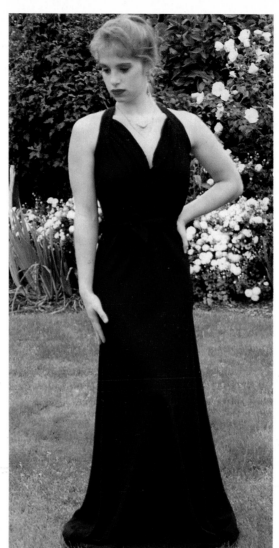

A satin evening gown featuring ruching along the neckline and sleeves. *Courtesy of The Very Little Theatre.*

A navy crepe evening gown with a plunging neckline and added interest at the back. *Courtesy of The Very Little Theatre.*

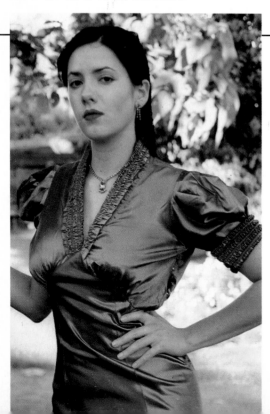

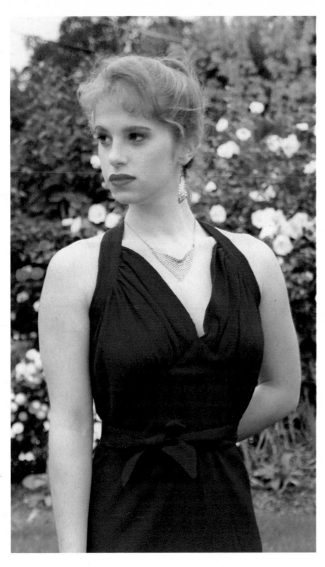

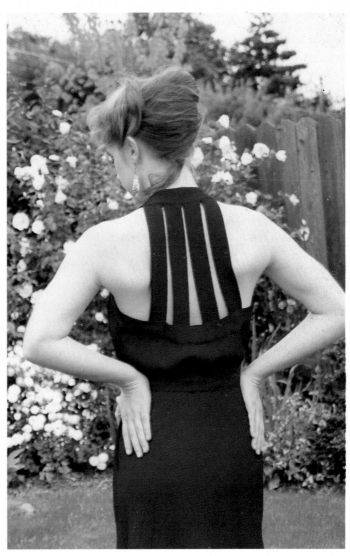

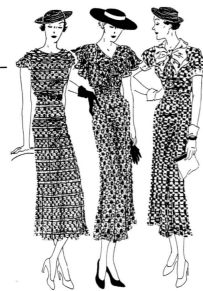

Three "everyday" dresses, featuring very typical drooping bows and narrow belts.

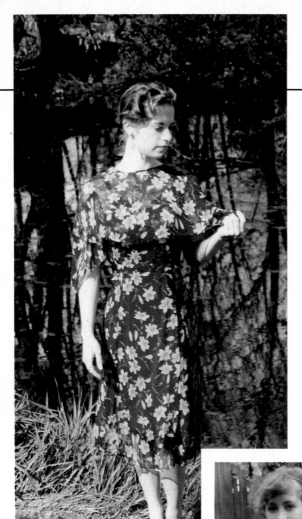

This soft, draped dress is of ultra–sheer printed chiffon. *Courtesy of The Very Little Theatre.*

Two "afternoon" dresses, as shown in the McCall Pattern Company catalog.

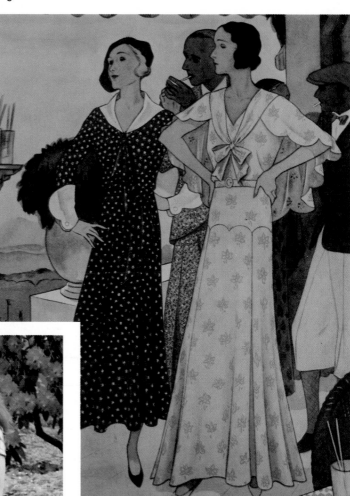

A circa 1937 neo-Victorian dress of colorful plaid, trimmed with lace.

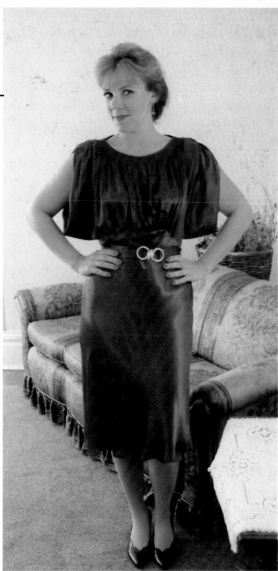

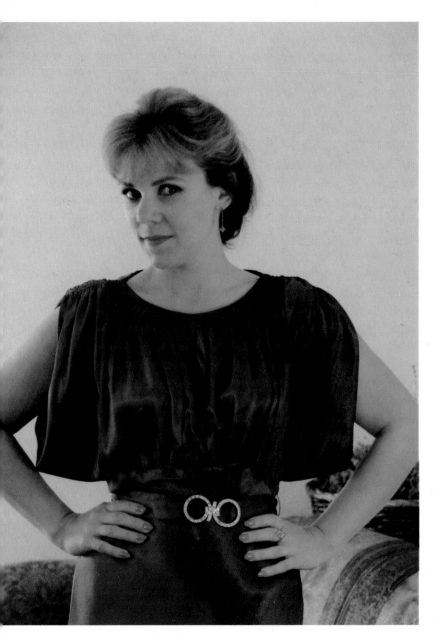

Ruching, a rhinestone belt clasp, and an unusual sleeve style are featured on this rich satin dress. *Courtesy of The Very Little Theatre.*

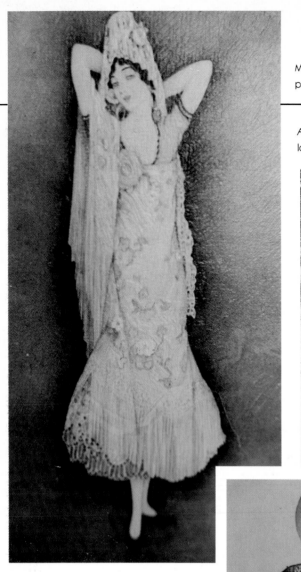

Many dresses continued to find inspiration from other cultures. This painting features an early thirties dress with Spanish influence.

A crepe evening gown designed to make long legs appear even longer. *Courtesy of The Very Little Theatre.*

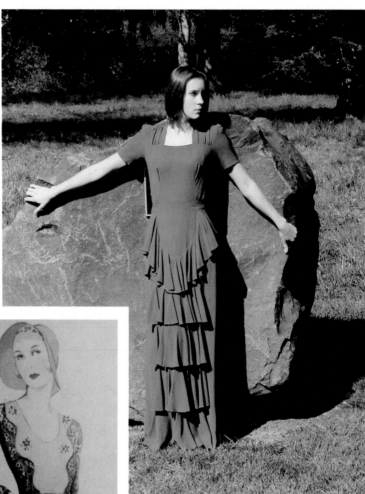

A practical and pretty ready-to-wear dress.

Summer day dresses from the McCall Pattern Company catalog.

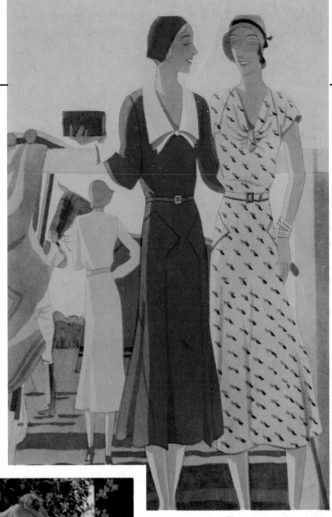

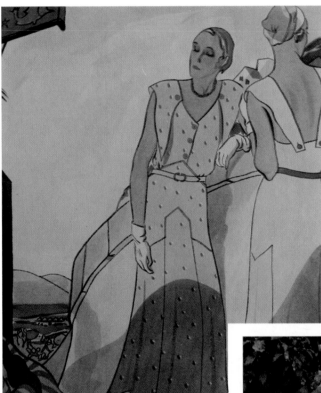

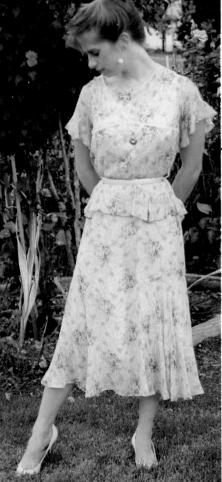

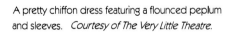

A pretty chiffon dress featuring a flounced peplum and sleeves. *Courtesy of The Very Little Theatre.*

A classic day dress of the thirties.

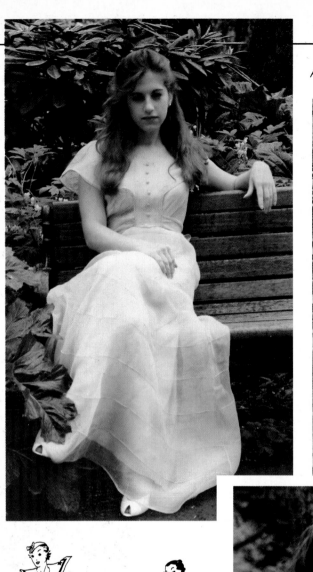

A romantic organdy dress. *Courtesy of The Very Little Theatre.*

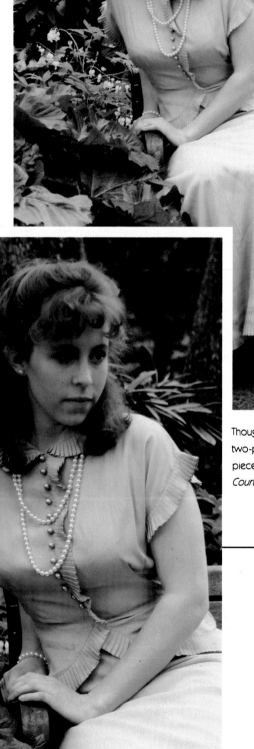

Daywear designs for the summer.

Though at first it appears to be two-piece, this classic is one-piece, trimmed subtlely with pleats. *Courtesy of The Very Little Theatre.*

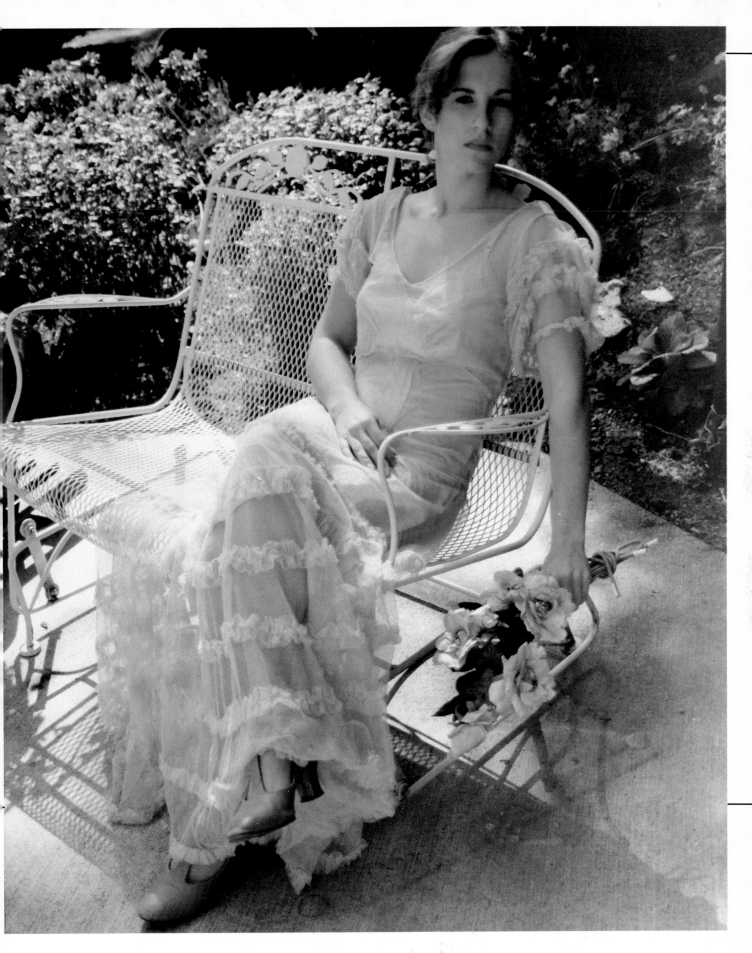

A dreamy sheer dress, frilled with flounces. *Courtesy of Marianine's Vintage Chic.*

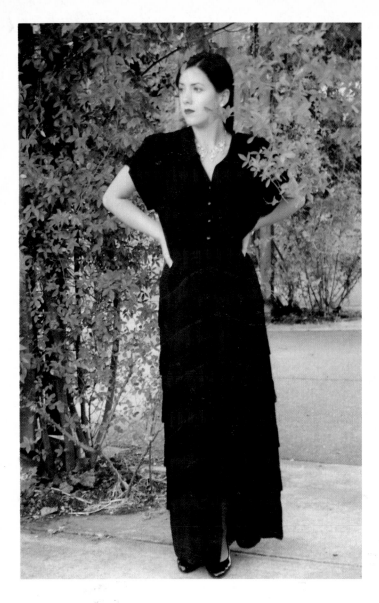

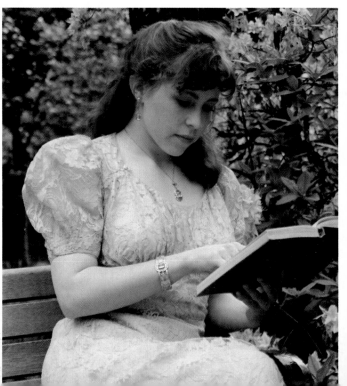

An evening dress featuring a fringe-trimmed skirt, circa 1939. *Courtesy of* The Very Little Theatre.

Lace dresses like these are abundantly available to collectors—they are bridesmaid dresses that were tucked away for safekeeping after the wedding. *Courtesy of* The Very Little Theatre.

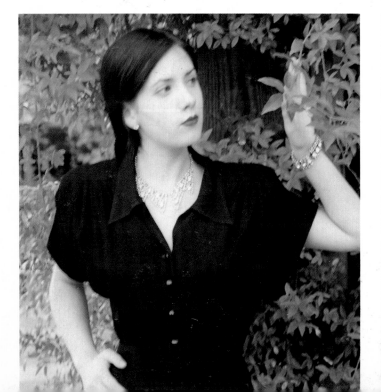

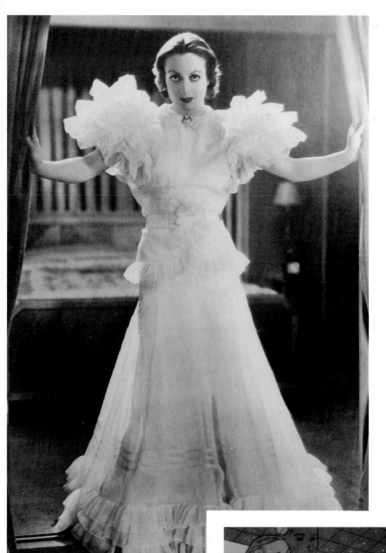

Movie actress Joan Crawford symbolized the woman of the era: lean, sophisticated, and bold.

This lace dress with a peplum-trimmed bolero dates to circa 1939–1940. *Courtesy of The Very Little Theatre.*

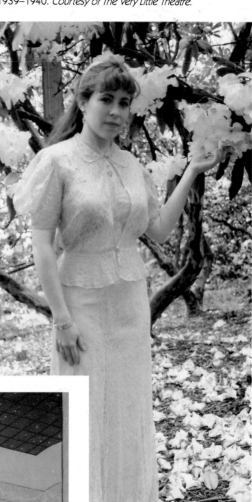

Though many dresses of the period were simple in line, their cut was sometimes on the complicated side, as this McCall Pattern Company pattern plate illustrates.

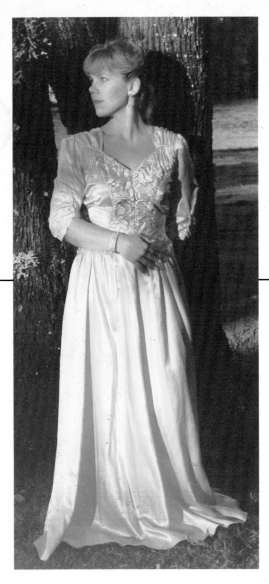

An especially rich satin evening gown featuring a sweetheart neckline and a ruched bodice.

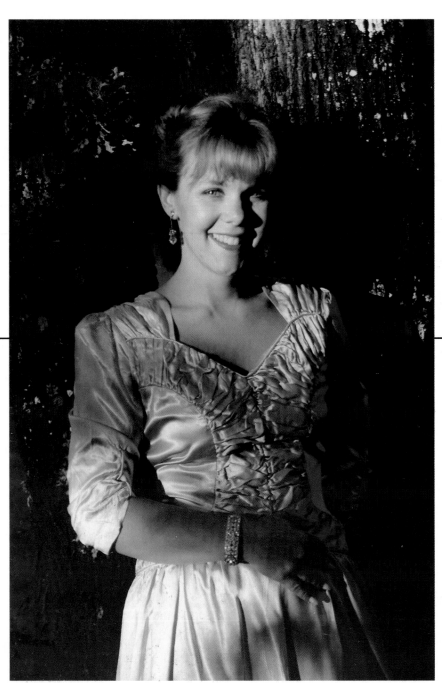

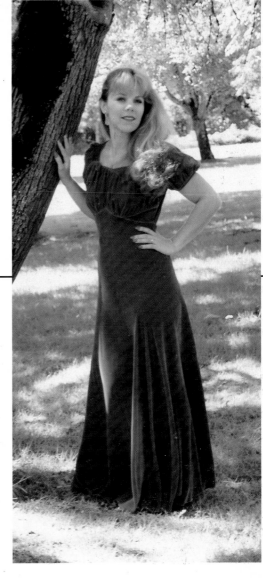

A silk velvet evening gown. *Courtesy of The Very Little Theatre.*

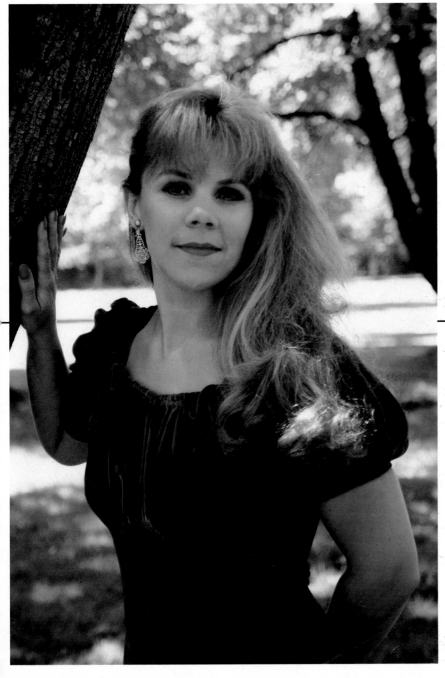

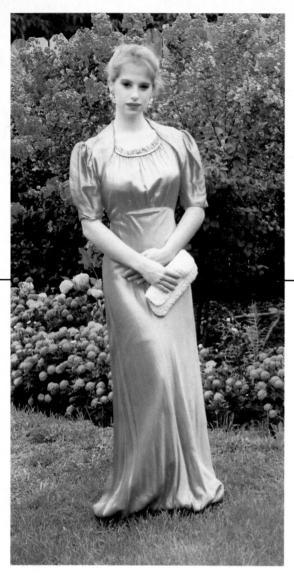

This satin evening gown features an interesting shoulder design and an attached "necklace" of rhinestones. *Courtesy of The Very Little Theatre.*

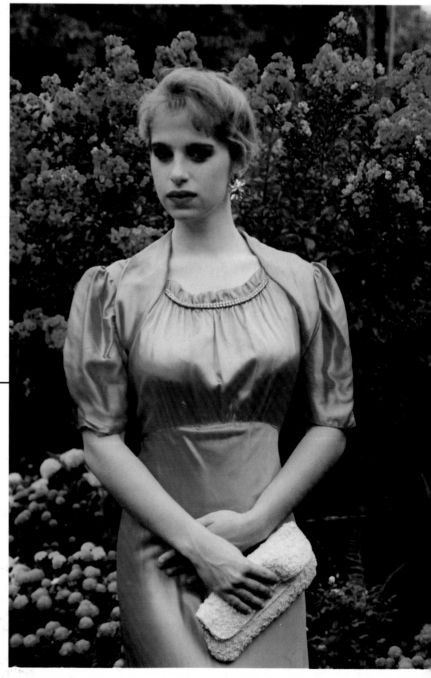

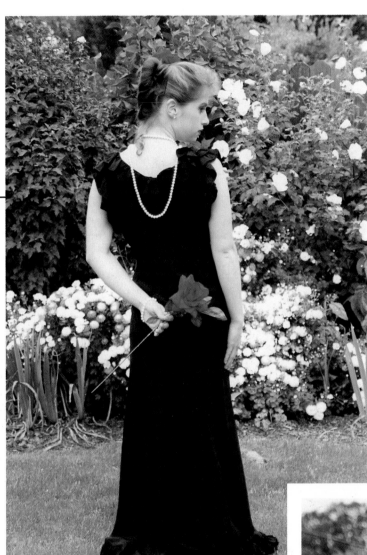

A little black evening gown trimmed with ruching. *Courtesy of The Very Little Theatre.*

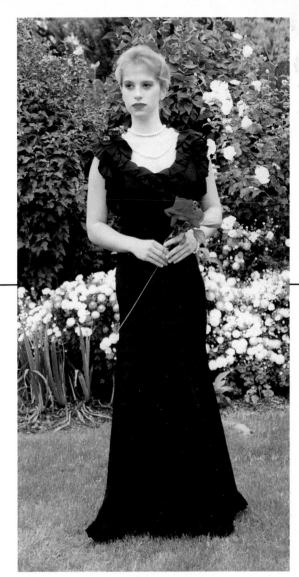

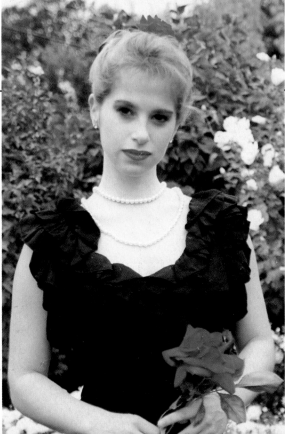

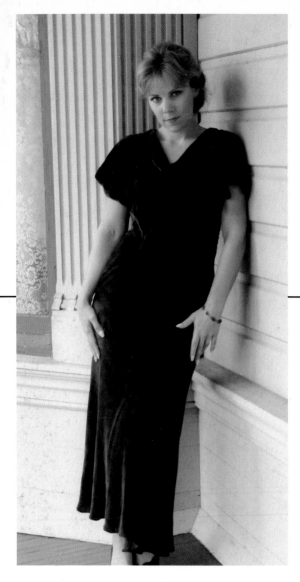

A typical velvet gown from the period, featuring a cowl neckline and scalloped sleeves. The garment label indicates it was made up in a patented fabric, but what was meant by "transparent," is unclear, since the fabric is hardly transparent. *Courtesy of The Very Little Theatre.*

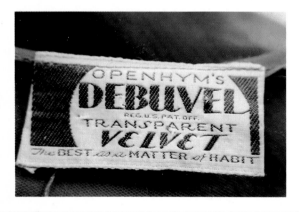

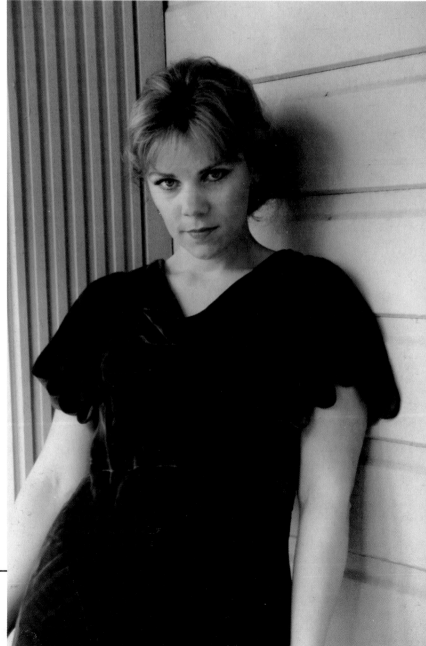

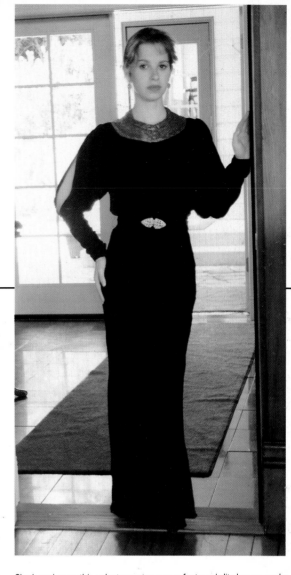

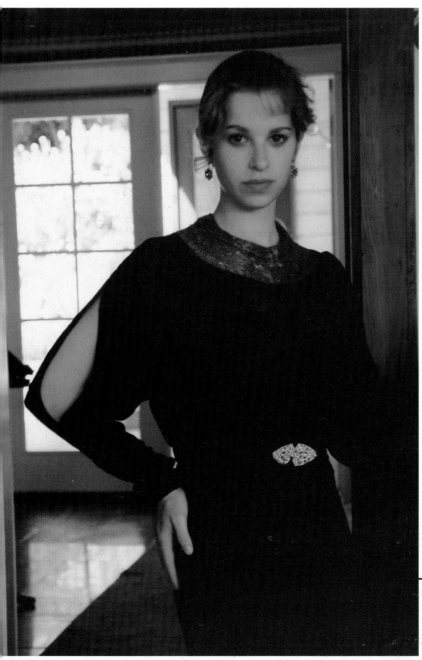

Sleek and sexy, this velvet evening gown featured slit sleeves and a cut metal collar. *Courtesy of Marianine's Vintage Chic.*

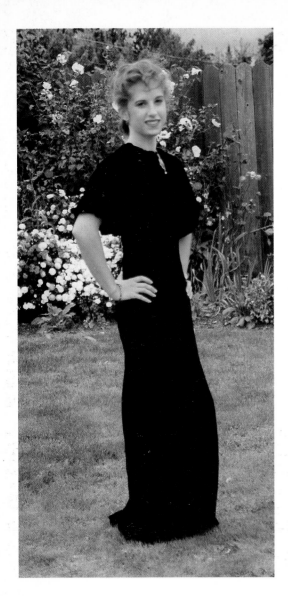

Velvet evening gowns from the thirties are relatively easy to find. This one stands out from the crowd with its full, balloon sleeves and ruff collar. *Courtesy of The Very Little Theatre.*

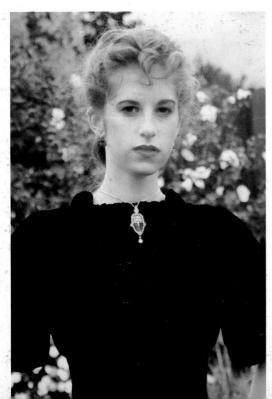

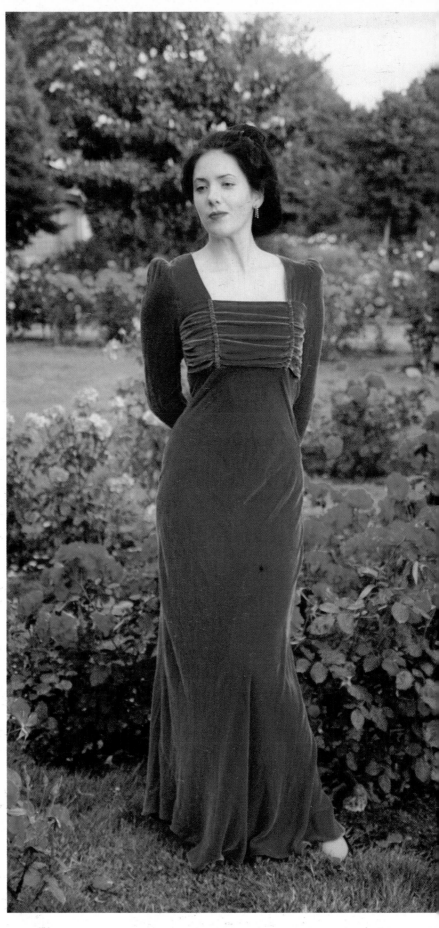

An exquisite royal blue velvet evening gown. *Courtesy of The Very Little Theatre.*

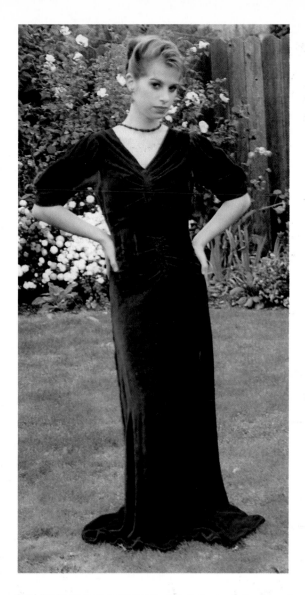

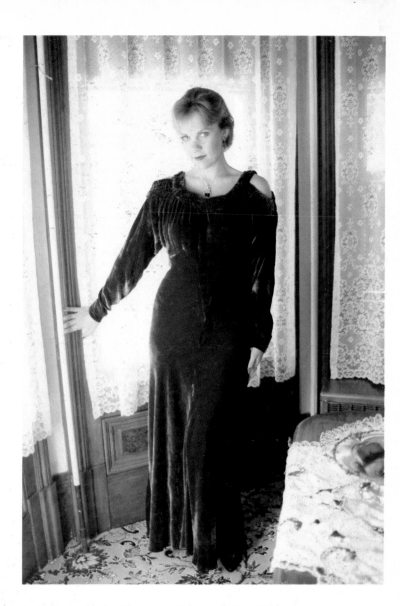

Carefully placed ruching makes this velvet gown novel. *Courtesy of The Very Little Theatre.*

A silk velvet evening gown featuring an unusual off–the–shoulder look. *Courtesy of The Very Little Theatre.*

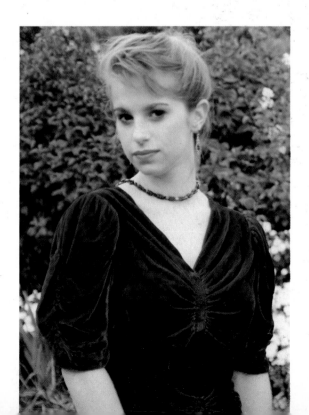

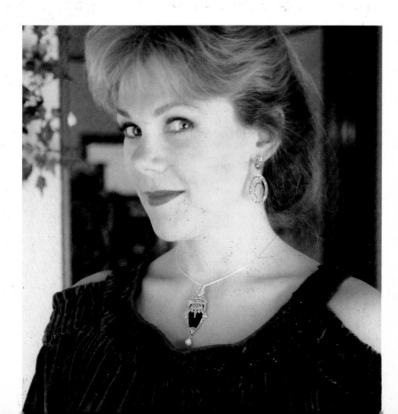

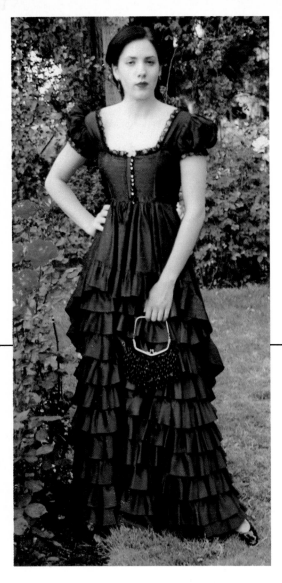

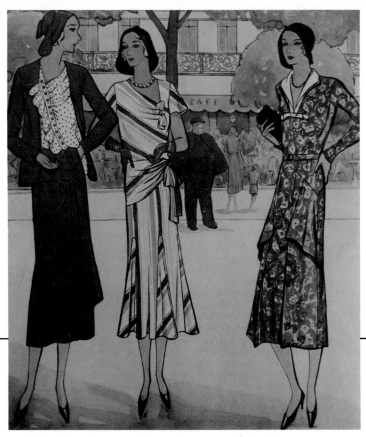

A typical thirties suit (at left), as featured in the McCall Pattern Company catalog. The skirt is perfectly plain and almost perfectly straight. The gaudy dress prints are typical of the era.

A neo-Victorian iridescent taffeta evening dress, featuring short, puff sleeves and abundant ruffles. *Courtesy of The Very Little Theatre.*

A dance-hall style evening gown of netting and lace, circa 1939–1940. *Courtesy of The Very Little Theatre.*

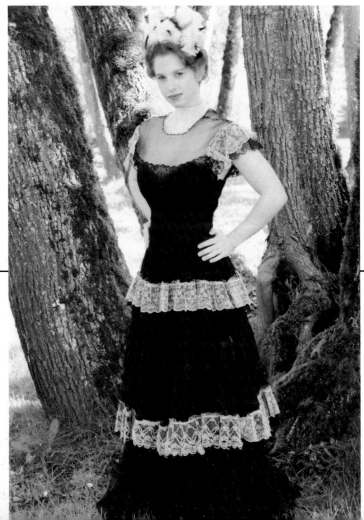

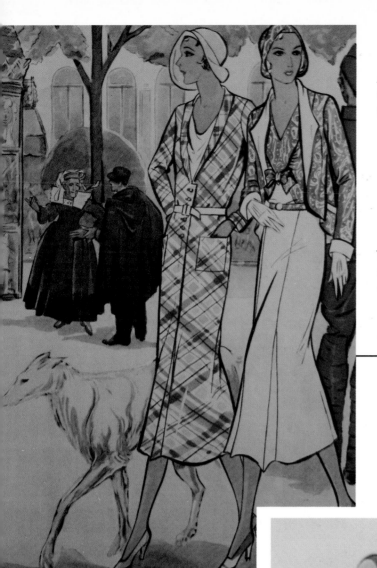

A more typical skirt, featuring pleats that begin just above the knee for ease in walking. Notice that even the one-piece dress is made to look like a suit.

No. 559
Size 18
36 Bust 39 Hip

HOLLYWOOD

PATTERN

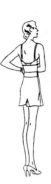

Typical underwear of the thirties, as illustrated on a Hollywood sewing pattern: bra and tap–pants.

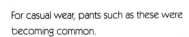

For casual wear, pants such as these were becoming common.

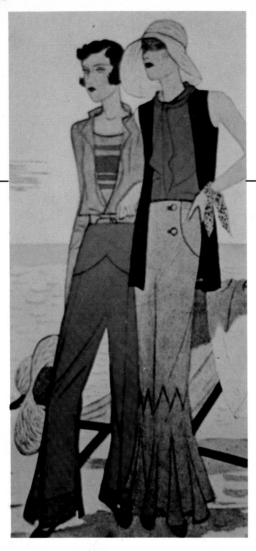

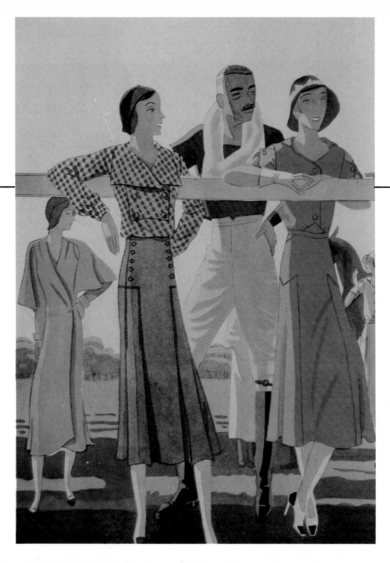

Most pants from the thirties are fitted at the hip, then flare (to varying widths) just below the knee.

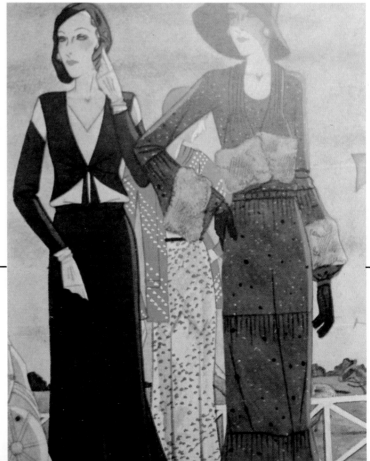

Typical skirt styles, as McCall's published them. The look was tailored and angular.

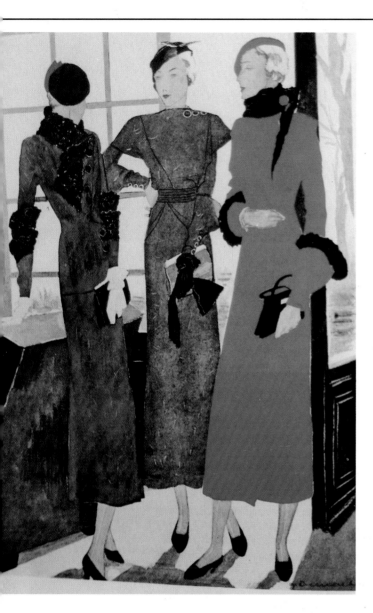

Fashionable coats of the thirties followed the same style lines as dresses, and often featured fur.

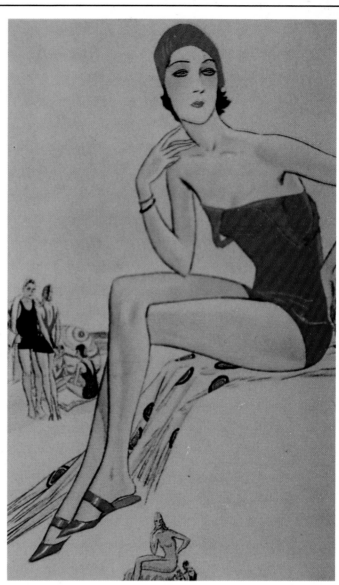

Vogue showcased minimal suits for sunbathing.

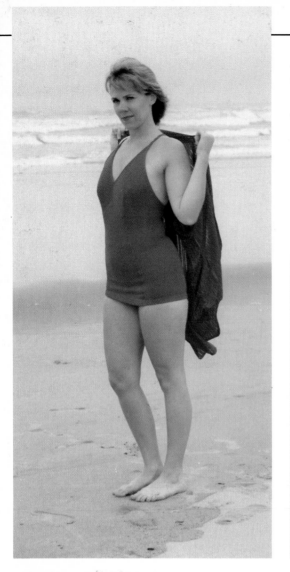

A bathing suit nearly identical to the one featured in *Vogue*, but manufactured by J.C. Penny. *Courtesy of The Very Little Theatre.*

A pillbox-type hat of draped velvet. *Courtesy of The Very Little Theatre.*

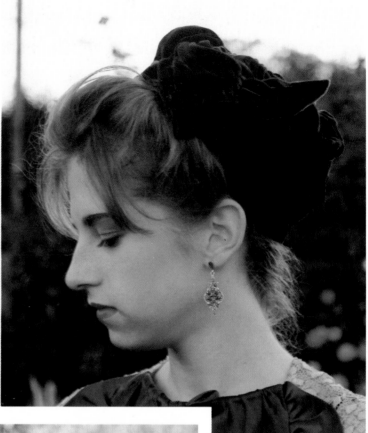

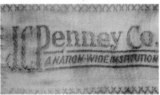

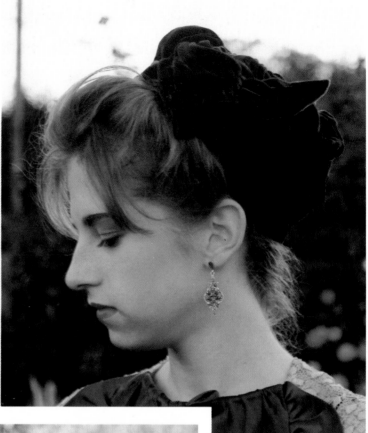

An "Empress Eugenie" hat. *Courtesy of The Very Little Theatre.*

From the late 1930s, turquoise printed shoes trimmed with gold and silver. *Courtesy of The Very Little Theatre.*

This "Empress Eugenie" hat is little more than feathers shaped like flowers circling the head. *Courtesy of The Very Little Theatre.*

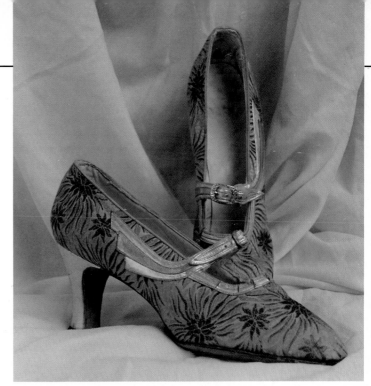

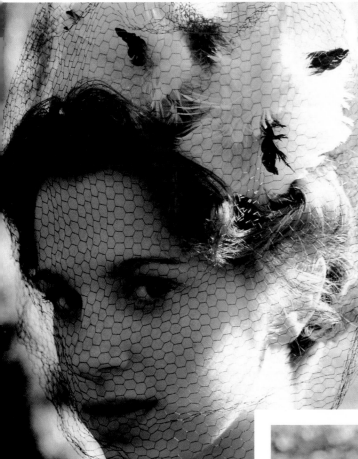

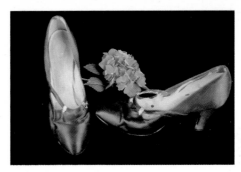

Iridescent shoes trimmed with rhinestones. *Courtesy of The Very Little Theatre.*

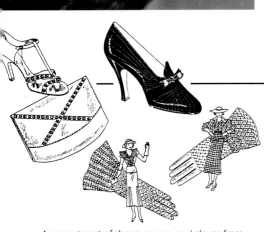

An assortment of shoes, purses, and gloves from the 1930s.

A tiny "Empress Eugenie" hat trimmed with fat plumes. *Courtesy of The Very Little Theatre.*

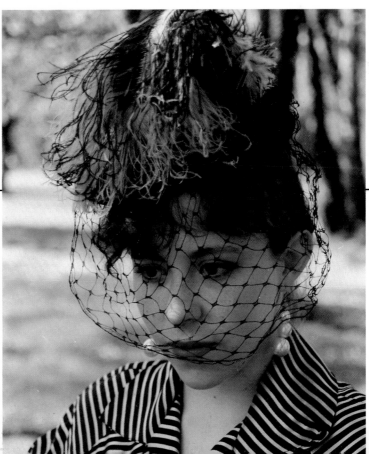

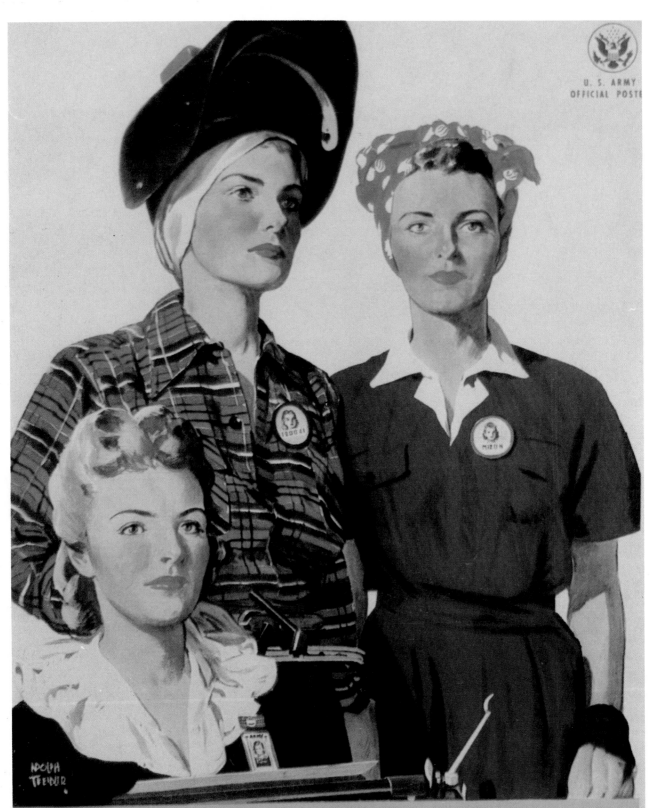

U. S. ARMY
OFFICIAL POSTE

SOLDIERS *without guns*

CHAPTER SIX

1940S: INDEPENDENT WOMAN

"Gee! I wish I were *a man*! I'd join the navy!" WWI recruiting posters headlined, picturing a coy, cute young woman in a sailor's guise. A far cry from WWII posters where the heroine Rosie the Riveter was pictured in drab blues, a scarf around her head, her sleeves rolled up. "We can do it!" Rosie exclaimed, her arm muscles flexed to prove it. "Soldiers *without* guns," another ad campaign dubbed the more than six million working American women (over half of whom had never worked outside the home before). Donning factory overalls in the daytime and feminine styles (to perk up "the boys") in the evening: this was the American woman's new job—what she considered her duty.

War rationings on fabrics put a sudden strain on the fashion industry's creativity. European designs became virtually impossible to import. American designers were still fledgling, and found it difficult to be taken seriously—so much so that their clothes infrequently carried their names; only the name of the company that manufactured the garment or the store that sold it appeared. Would fashion survive?

"Shortages, rationings, taxes, actual war losses . . ." *Mademoiselle* speculated in 1942, "will the new restrictions hamper the creativeness of American designers (and where else save in America can fashions be designed any more)? Can women be both chic and patriotic? [Women] are wanting something practical . . . something feminine. Women can help win a war by just being women, you know!" Fashion magazines all over the United States did their best to convince women that buying new clothing was the right thing to do—that it helped support the economy, and would help the United States win the war. And, indeed, not only did women continue to buy clothing, but by the end of the decade, they had made the American designer supreme.

By looking at rationing and restrictions not as hindrances but as challenges, American designers (both famous and anonymous) created a fresh, pleasing look for the era. So much so, in fact, that *Collier's* soon proclaimed that "American women are the best dressed in the world!" American ready-to-wear designers also made new strides in their ever-growing industry, fleshing out sizing standards, and including fiber content and care labels for the first time.

Other fashion segments also flourished. While the War Production Board initiated restrictions to strictly dictate how wide and long a woman's skirt should be, it allowed infants' and toddlers' apparel, maternity dresses, and bridal gowns to be totally exempt from their mandates.

Furthermore, the home-sewing industry continued to flourish; paper pattern and needlework tool sales were at an all-time high. While the Victorian woman felt blessed that her treadle sewing machine could sew 1,477 stitches a minute, the new electric sewing machine boasted a previously unheard-of 3,000 stitches per minute.

DRESSES

"Woman's figure is the exclamation point of the world," author Carrie Hall wrote of then-current Forties styles. "Today there is an absence of curves." This may have been due, at least in part, to the continuing style of "made-over" clothes. Though many women had for at least a decade steadily refashioned their clothes, women of the forties found a new resource: the suits their husbands, fathers, and brothers left behind when they went to war. Made up in fine woolens, its no wonder many women cut up such suits and refashioned them into styles they could wear. Even ready-to-wear suits (which were, for the first time, in real competition with dresses) were advertised as "man-tailored"—implying that they were sturdy and practical.

Most often, such suits were boxy, with narrow skirts, wide shoulders, and barely nipped–in waists. For the vast number of new working women, suits were indispensable. As Carrie Hall wrote, "The business woman, above all others, should wear nothing that attracts more attention than her personality, otherwise the value of her ego will be lost." Even in the evening, suits were the new staple, made more glamorous by the use of velvets and metallics, with beaded accents and rhinestone buttons.

Previous page:
Government campaigns during World War II convinced women they could be independent.

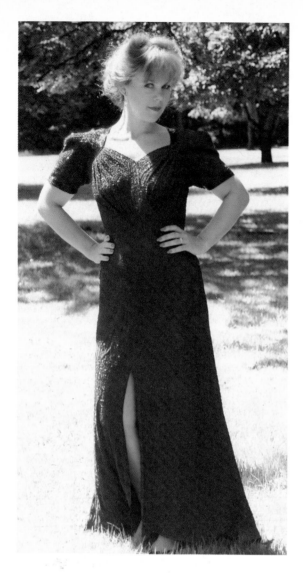

An evening dress with an all-over beaded design. *Courtesy of The Very Little Theatre.*

By day, however, dresses were generally more casual than they had ever been. Dresses from Mexico soon became popular because they were inexpensive and colorful, and within a few years American manufacturers began imitating Mexican and other ethnic styles. Perhaps because women were suddenly required to dig up their old pioneering spirit, Western styles also rushed into fashion, as did gingham "pioneer" looks. *Harper's Bazaar* tried to convince their readers of the economy and fun of these modes: "Play with the fruits of a journey . . . Girls are bringing back frontier pants from the general store in Saskachewan. Buckskin jackets from Alaska. A bright pink rebozo or a rampantly sequined *ching poblana* skirt from Mexico. A Daniel Boone fur hat from Banff . . . a poncho from the Argentine . . ."

Despite all this "good old-fashioned" style, women clung to modern conveniences. By now, most dresses were fastened with a zipper (though until circa 1947, it continued to run up the side of the dress, not straight down the back). However, *Harper's* had warnings that indicated many women were indiscreet about their "zips:" "No lady shows her zippers . . . Zippers are as private as yawns or stays or garters. They should be used, but not seen."

Rayon—the modern miracle—was easily the most popular fabric used in dresses, and though woolens were still favored for suits, both wool and silk were in short supply during the war. Instead, women of the forties chose gabardine for suits, and crepes and failles for other dresses. Single color dresses were favored by day—black being *the* color, by day or night. Suits, on the other hand, could be plain, or full of checks, stripes, or plaids.

"It's the American way to live in a dress with a jacket!" Sears catalog stated, and indeed, a simple day dress worn with a well-tailored suit jacket was just the thing when a tailored but slightly softer look was preferred. By 1945, however, *Vogue* magazine complained about this boxy, tailored look. "The way not to look this year is hard, sharp, cold, even bold," they explained. "It's out because the men can't bear it." Similarly, *Mademoiselle* spoke against what had became the popular wearing of uniforms. "A uniform," the editors insisted, "should be as *deserved* by the woman who wears it as by the soldier who wears one. And even so, she should still wear it only in her line of duty. When a soldier goes out with his girl, or his wife, or his mother, he wants—and needs—undisguised femininity."

Thus long, feminine dresses still reigned at night, and beaded dresses were still fashionable. Sequins, however, were the queen of the evening. Unlike many other materials, sequins weren't rationed (though some joked they might be used to blind the enemy), and they soon became a simple and inexpensive way to add some sparkle to evening wear.

Skirts & Slacks

Nowhere were war restrictions more noticeable than they were in skirts: No wider than 72 to 80 inches (according to the size of the finished garment), no ruffles or flounces, no hems any wider than two inches. However, such restrictions only applied to the ready-to-wear and couture industries, since it was impossible for the government to regulate home-sewers (though most home-sewers would have wanted to be patriotic and therefore somewhat frugal). Still, by the early forties, skirts were easily knee length and did not drop one iota until about 1945, when a slightly longer look prevailed.

Though most skirts were narrow and boxy, when restrictions were not applicable so-called "sunburst" skirts, pleated entirely around their circumference, were popular. Broom skirts (those long and fashionably wrinkled gems) also first appeared

138

in the forties, and were so dubbed because they were "crinkled" by wrapping them while wet around a broomstick, and tying them thus with string until they dried.

Still, if you ask many women who lived through the 1940s what they wore most often, chances are they'll say unequivocally: "Pants." Yes, slacks had finally "made it." Worn by day in the fitted torso, slightly bell–bottomed style, even fashion magazines featured them regularly in their pages. And as women became prominent in the workplace, pants became more than just fashionable—they were essential.

This new, feminine influence upon the workplace sent many business owners scrambling. Much talk was given about to how to deal with women on the job; most "experts" agreed that to keep a woman employee happy, you had to make sure her work uniform was attractive. As the July 1943 issue of *Mass Transportation Magazine* instructed managers of bus systems, women employees required a whole new set of rules:

> There's no longer any question whether transit companies should hire women for jobs formerly held by men. The draft and manpower shortage has settled that point. The important things now are how to select the most efficient women available and how to use them to the best advantage...Give every girl an adequate number of rest periods during the day. You have to make some allowances for feminine psychology. A girl has more confidence and is more efficient if she can keep her hair tidied, apply fresh lipstick and wash her hands several times a day...Get enough size variety in operators uniforms so that each girl can have a proper fit. This point can't be stressed too strongly as a means of keeping women happy...

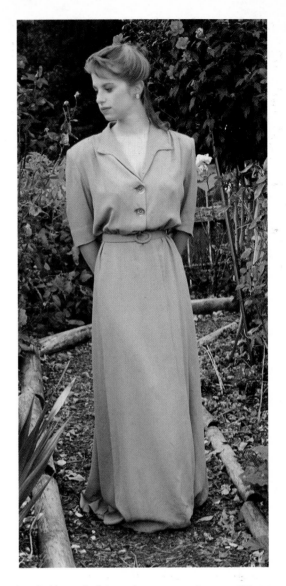

A typical "everyday" dress of rayon crepe. *Courtesy of The Very Little Theatre.*

BLOUSES

Shoulder pads were the predominant feature in blouses of the 1940s. No blouse could be considered really fashionable unless it had pads that gave a fat, hard, shelf–like edge to the shoulders (unlike the softly-shaped shoulder pads of the thirties).

But shoulder pads were the only frivolity allowed. Rationing restrictions kept blouses simple—and not infrequently, totally plain. Though a single blouse pocket was allowed, more than one was starkly against restrictions.

Sweaters, on the other hand, seemed to grow more elaborate. Whether made at home or purchased ready–made, sweaters were popular in nearly every fabric imaginable (the most expensive being cashmere), and were often decorated with carnival glass or other types of beads.

LEISURE WEAR

The sundresses and pants outfits of the 1930s remained popular for casual wear in the forties, but alongside these staples the "play suit" emerged. These girlish outfits commonly featured a sleeveless top worn with a skirt that buttoned up the front; beneath the skirt, bloomer-like shorts that ended at the upper thigh were worn, and could be revealed by unfastening several of the skirt's buttons. Such outfits became increasingly popular at the beach, while picnicking, or gardening, until they too became fashion staples in the next decade.

Having been extremely simple for some time, bathing suits finally took a new turn. No longer were completely trim–free, figure–hugging suits favored. The new style was feminine: sweetheart necklines, ruched trim, scant skirts or flounces at the hip. As the bustline became increasingly important, Jantzen intro-

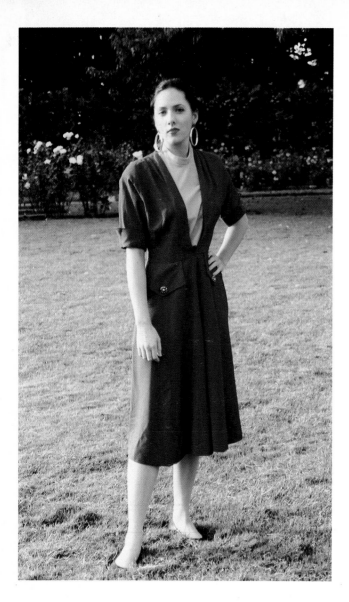

A day dress of denim–colored cotton and silver buttons. The yellow "V" in front is actually a jersey dickey. *Courtesy of The Very Little Theatre.*

duced the "Beauty–Life Bra" built into their suits. Other ingenious beauty aids were also hidden: tummy– and hip–flattening girdles, elasticized shoulder straps, and gentle waist–nippers. By 1949, the strapless swimsuit became the latest in fashion, making men ponder why the suit didn't fall down, and women worry how long it would manage to stay up. Two–piece bathing suits (modest by later twentieth century standards, but said in the Forties to "reveal everything about a girl except her mother's maiden name") were steadily pushed by bathing suit manufacturers. Still, the wearing of them was by no means universal. "Why, they come off in the water," movie mermaid Esther Williams complained. "If you can't swim in them, what good are they?"

LINGERIE

The lingerie of the 1940s is an area that is largely unexplored by most collectors. While slips and other basic undergarments remained much the same in the forties as they had been in the previous decade (though they tended to be more snug), there were some interesting changes in lingerie.

The bra, for instance, really came into its own in the forties. From the strapless (and often backless) "Merry Widow" style that reached all the way down to the waist, to the first wired "full-figure" bras, to the first "bullet bras" (quilted and shaped in a most exaggerated form), the world of lingerie would never be the same again. For the first time since the turn of the century, bras and other "essentials" became decorative. Gone were the days of shapeless, simple chemises; the new lingerie was figure-hugging (often figure-forming), and embellished with laces and trims.

There was also another first in lingerie: though nylon stockings had only just been introduced in the late 1930s, it wasn't long before the newly discovered fabric was being rationed because of the war. But women didn't give up the better-fitting stockings easily. "There was a feverish and unremitting pursuit of nylons," Carrie Hall wrote. "A rumor that a store had received a consignment would conjure up queues thousands long for a small stock that would melt away in minutes." Normally, only one pair was allowed per customer, so women enlisted their young sons and daughters to stand in line with them, to pick up extra pairs.

Nonetheless, many women were forced to go without. Rather than don old-fashioned and uncomfortable rayon stockings, many women went bare-legged—a state for which cosmetic manufacturers quickly developed a product: Special make-up to simulate nylons—from the all-over tan/nude color right down to the seam running down the back of the leg. Fashion magazines offered another solution: a new mode for wearing socks (even with dresses), either knee- or ankle-length.

OTHER IMPORTANT GARMENTS

Hats were essential to the forties look, often worn over decorative hairnets called snoods (a fashion stolen from Civil War–era ancestors). Though women's clothes were eminently practical, hats were exceptionally outlandish. Decorated with ribbon remnants, feathers (and actual birds), beading, and any other oddball trim that was on hand, hats were the fun part of dressing. Bits of netting could be swathed on top, or dropped down mysteriously over the eyes. Hats became everything from pillbox-like wisps to top hat–style monstrosities. For more casual events, a practical turban or headscarf might be worn instead.

Shoes also made the news, ranging from platform styles (where the entire sole was thick, and the heel was down–right fat), to "wedgies" (which eliminated the shoes' arch and created only one long, ever–fattening, thick sole). In some cases, both leather and steel were rationed, really making designers rely on creativity. Cork was often used for soles (especially for "wedgies"), and in Europe, the early form of plastic called Bakelite was favored. In all cases, shoes were clunky, thickly soled (typically one to two inches thick), and often had ankle straps.

The "New Look"

In 1947, after World War II was over, couture designer Christian Dior launched a thoroughly refreshing fashion campaign. Using the nipped waists and long skirts that had been briefly popular in 1939 (only to be dispelled when the war broke out), Dior embellished, trimmed, and feminized fashions in neo-Victorian style. After the rationings and restrictions of the war years, women gleefully accepted his full skirts worn over lightweight Civil War–style hoopskirts or crinolines, peplums, shaped waistbands, and frills. That same year, even down-to-earth fashion sources like the Sears catalog featured fashions in the new couture-inspired style. *Vogue* reveled in the femininity of it all: "From the era of Madame Bovary . . . wasp-waisted Gibson Girl shirtwaists, pleated or tucked . . . slow-sloped, easy shoulders . . . wrapped and bound middles—barrel (almost hobble) skirts—longer, deeply shaped shadow–box décolleté—padded hips . . ."

Gone were padded shoulders. Gone were boxy skirts. Gone were all "lines" and "angles." The New Look was the look of curves. "Corset" was no longer a dirty word; a mere five to six inches deep, the new corset—while it nipped inches off the waist—was more elastic than boning, and was worn over a long, slenderizing girdle. Hips could be padded with special "panniers" reminiscent of those worn in the eighteenth century. Bustles made of deeply pleated taffeta could be added under skirts. Push-up bras and crinoline petticoats reigned.

By night, strapless evening gowns with fitted waists and long, full skirts with trains were the new mode. By day, the look featured full, swinging skirts with tucked and ruffled blouses, worn with white gloves and a hat. Everything was splendid and frivolous—and it was more than just a fad. The New Look, though it was introduced and embraced late in the forties, would be the look of the decade to come.

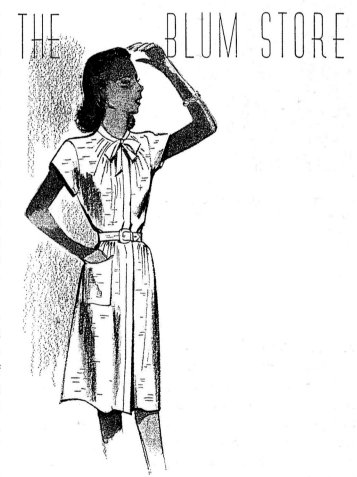

THE BLUM STORE

The new and ever-practical day dress, showcased in an advertisement by the Blum department store: rayon shantung, in "lime, aqua, melon pink! Sun-glow shades to light up your tan . . . show off the soft bow, brief sleeves, neat-nipped waist. Fly-front that speeds dressing time leads into skirt pleat."

141

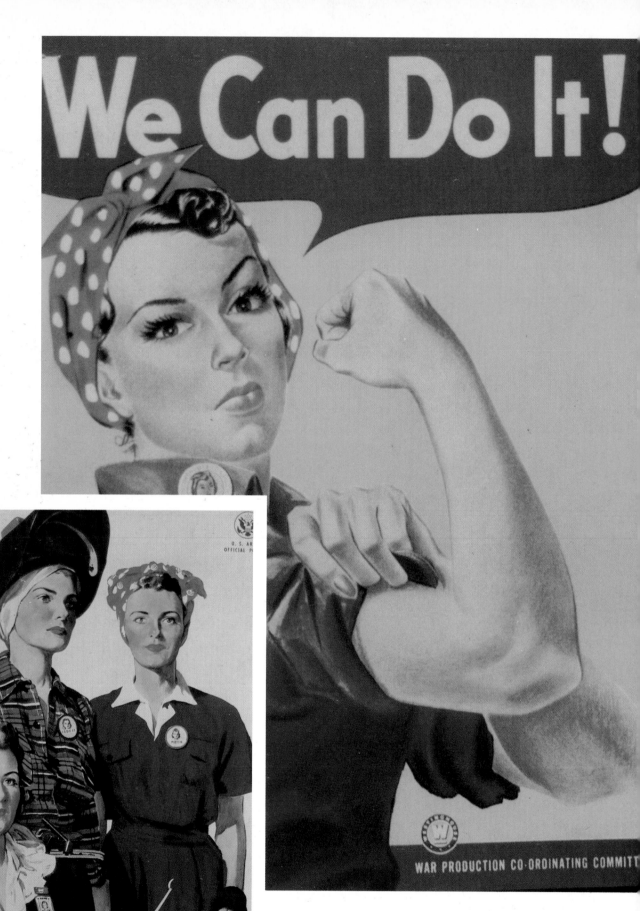

Two World War II posters, Rosie the Riveter style. The government did its best to convince women they could be independent—and it worked.

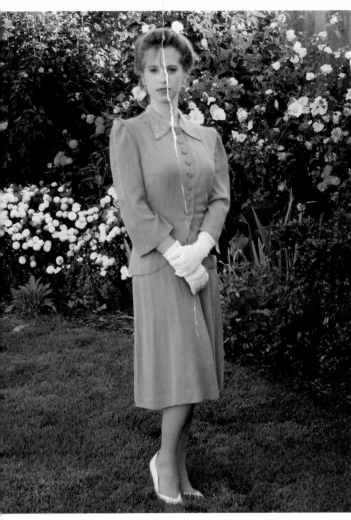

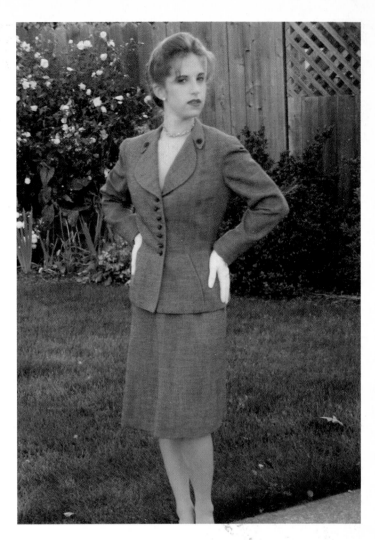

This soft suit with a beaded collar has only minimally padded shoulders—dating it to circa 1939–1940. *Courtesy of The Very Little Theatre.*

Clean, simple, and refined, this suit features small oblong buttons and short hip pockets. *Courtesy of The Very Little Theatre.*

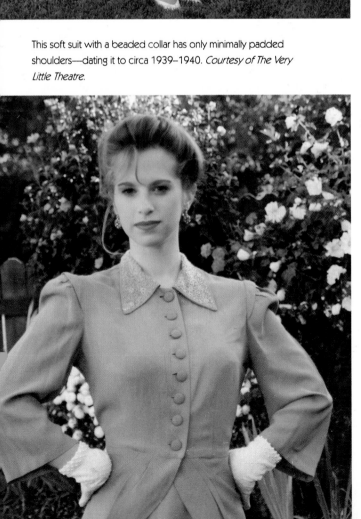

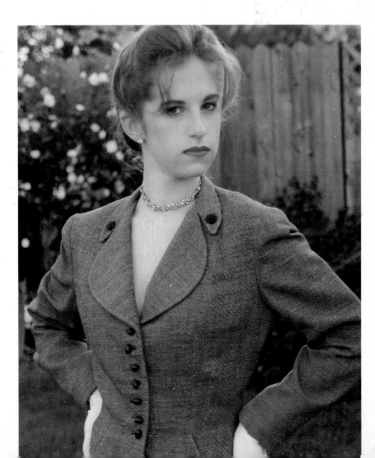

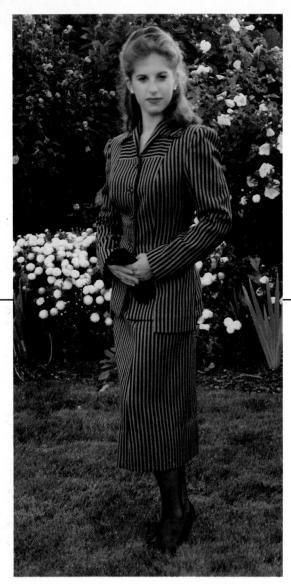

A stunning suit which uses stripes to their best advantage. The label is a good example of the usual inclusion of a department store or boutique label, but no designer label. *Courtesy of The Very Little Theatre.*

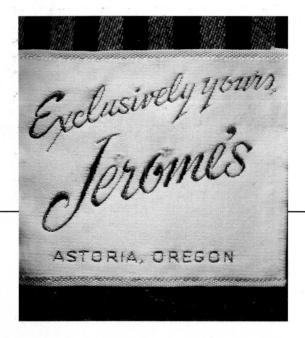

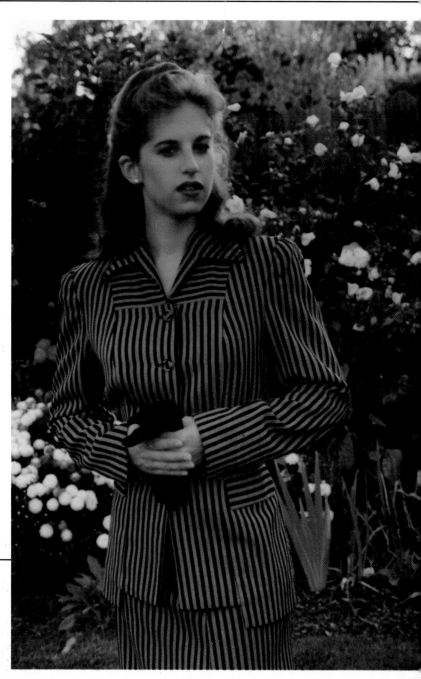

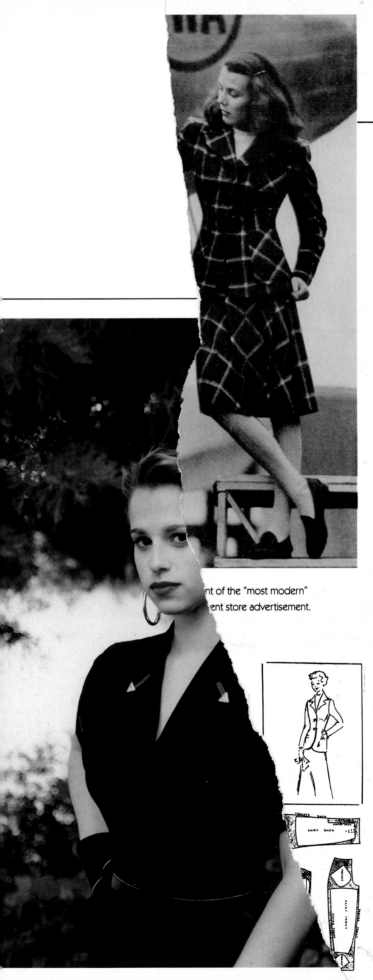

...nt of the "most modern"
...ent store advertisement.

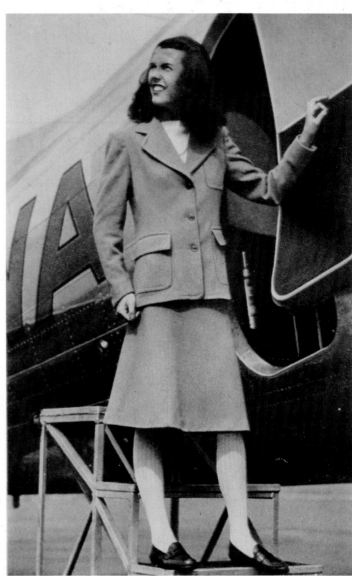

A basic suit, as featured in a 1941 Lord & Taylor department store advertisement.

For those who could not afford to go out and buy a new suit, sewing books and magazines of the period overflowed with clever ways to re–make old clothes. This diagram from *The Encyclopedia of Modern Sewing* (published in 1943) clearly illustrates how to take apart a man's suit and re–cut to fit a woman, and is an excellent example of the kind of economy many World War II women practiced.

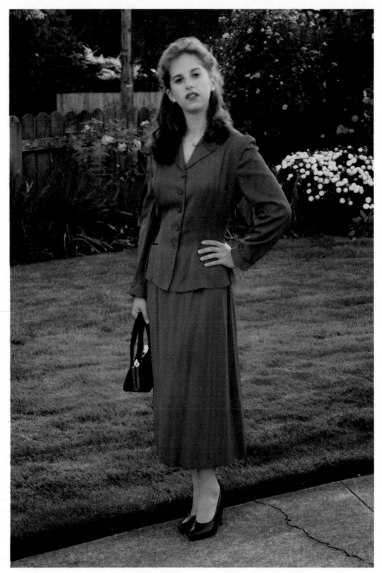

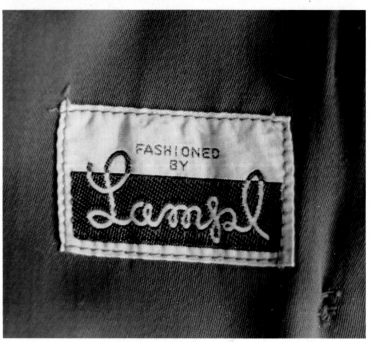

This rayon suit is cut with a slightly fuller skirt. *Courtesy of The Very Little Theatre.*

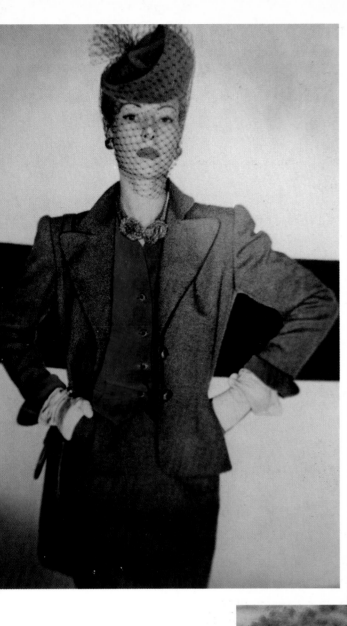

A debonair suit, featuring wine-colored velvet cuffs and a matching vest and hat.

Ladies' Home Journal featured what they called the "*big suit* in checked tweed with a box–pleated skirt" in their August 1948 issue.

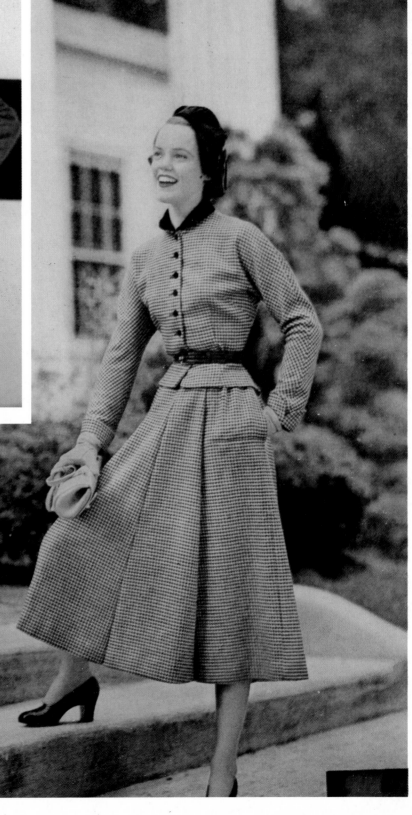

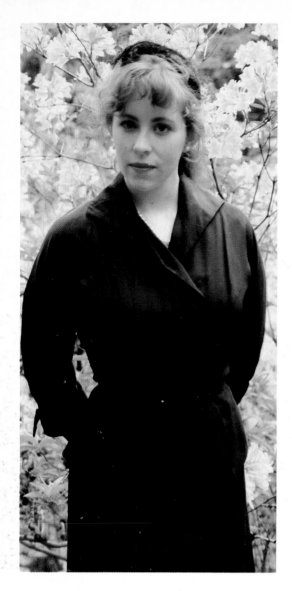

Notice the interesting "petal" cut on the peplum of this navy suit.
Courtesy of The Very Little Theatre.

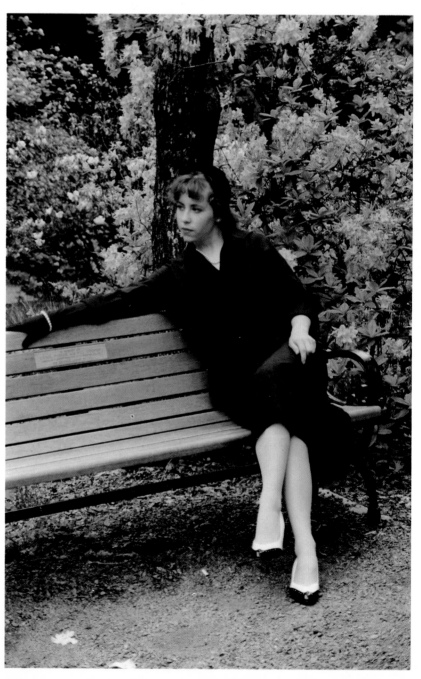

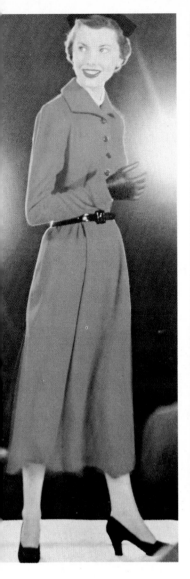
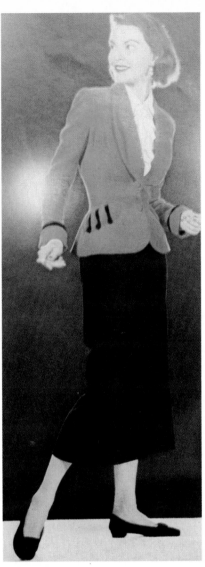
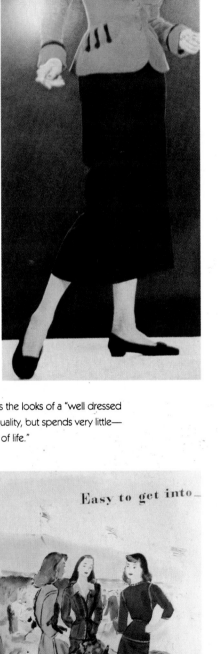

In 1949, *Glamour* described these as the looks of a "well dressed girl . . . She is the girl . . . Who buys quality, but spends very little—who falls for only what suits her way of life."

A striking wool suit from a Cerey Wools advertisement in 1949.

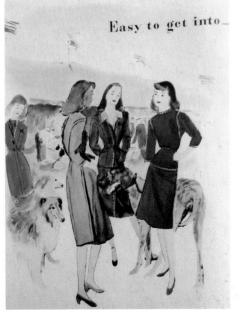

"Easy to get into!" This 1941 *Harper's Bazaar* layout stressed ease, comfort, and practicality.

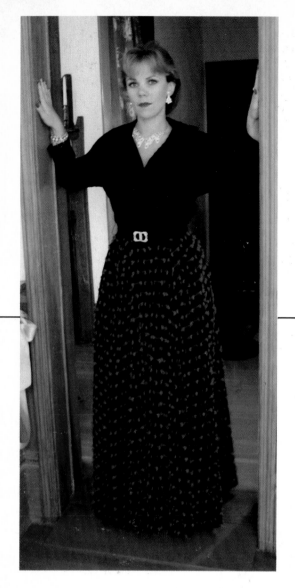

This classic forties "dinner dress" features a velvet bodice with a wide, pointed collar, and a taffeta skirt with red tufts swathing it.

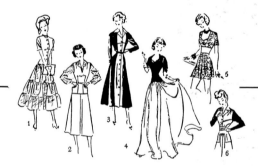

More re-styling ideas from *The Encyclopedia of Modern Sewing* (these from the 1947 edition): adding layers or ruffles to a too-short or tight skirt; making a jumper out of a shirt with wear on the sleeves; adding a contrasting panel to a too–small dress; adding a new, more fashionable bodice to an old dress; making a playsuit from a dress that is too short; and updating old shoulders with contrasting fabric and a revised design.

A "crisp embossed piqué in a one-piece, buttoned classic. Plunging neckline, kimono sleeves," said *The Ladies' Home Journal* of this 1949 Vogue Pattern design.

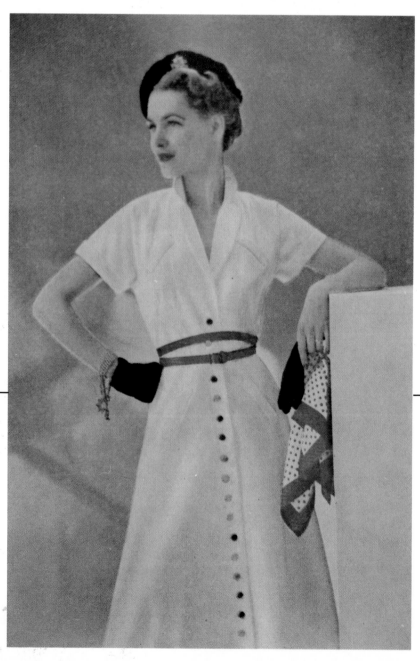

A laquered satin evening dress from circa 1947, featuring a soft peplum/bustle, graceful, sloping kimono sleeves, and (at last!) a zipper running down the back. *Courtesy of The Very Little Theatre.*

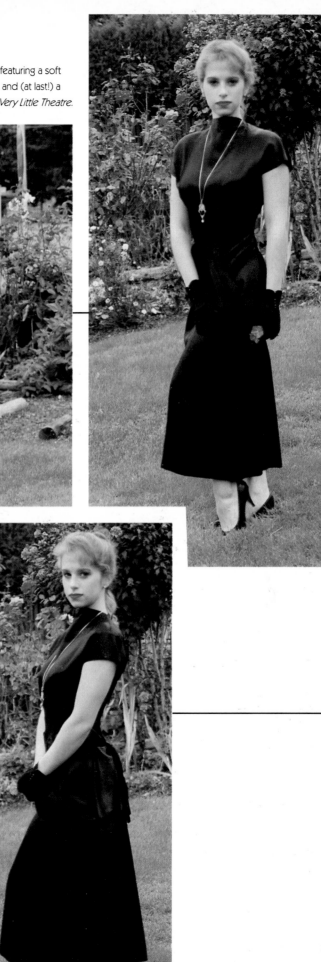

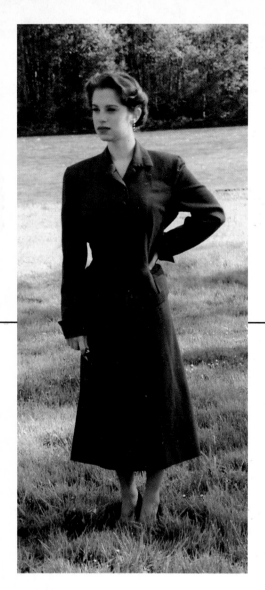

A burgundy wool suit. *Courtesy of The Very Little Theatre.*

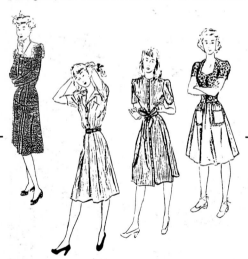

Everyday basics of the 1940s woman, as featured in the June 1942 issue of *Mademoiselle*: a rayon two-piece suit, a shirtwaist dress, a crisp chambray button-down dress, and a hand-crocheted sweater worn with a rayon skirt.

In 1945, as featured in a J. L. F. Originals advertisement, plaids were at the height of popularity, and bustles were making a modest debut.

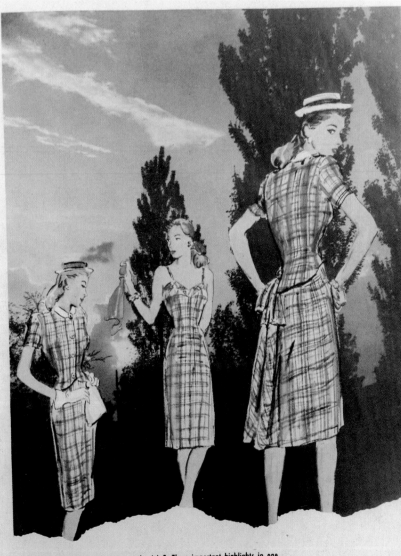

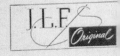

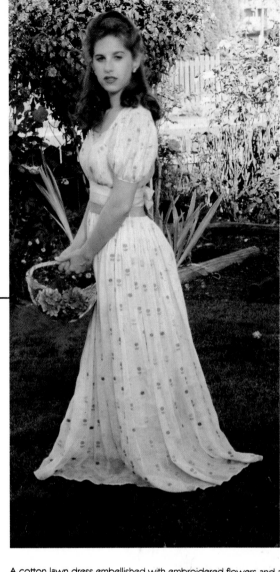

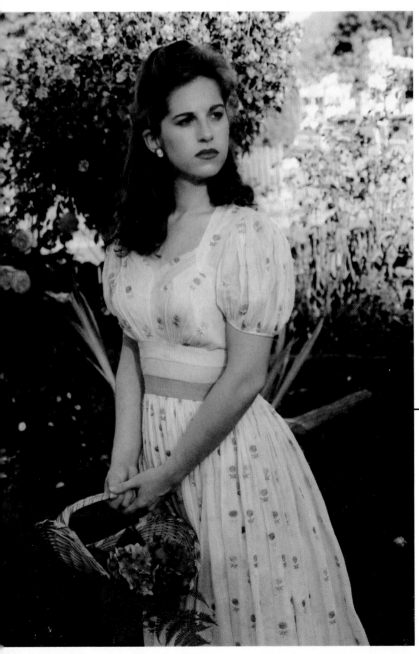

A cotton lawn dress embellished with embroidered flowers and a tri–ribbon waistband, circa 1947.

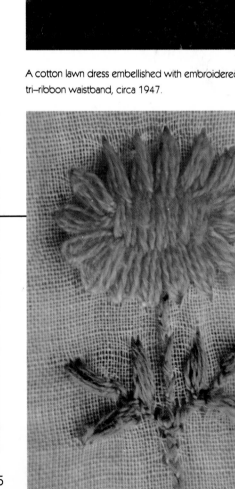

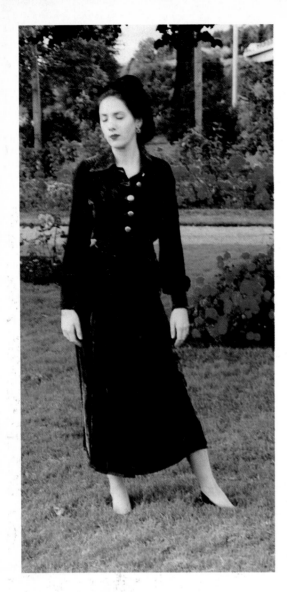

A rich silk velvet "dinner dress" garnished with smocking at the waist, collar, and cuffs. *Courtesy of The Very Little Theatre.*

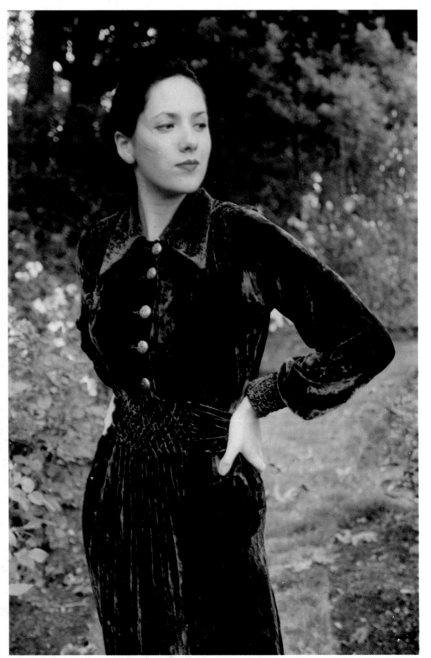

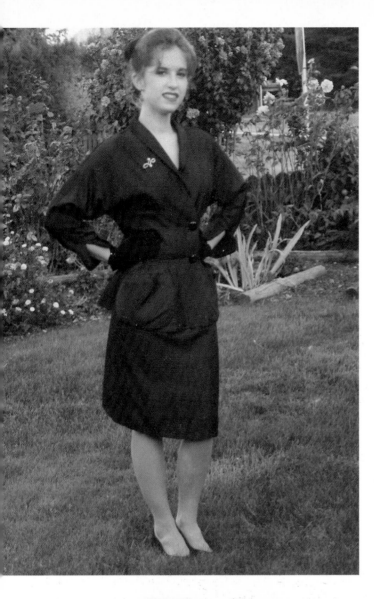

An iridescent wine-colored taffeta evening suit. *Courtesy of The Very Little Theatre.*

A chic wool felt dress from circa 1948. *Courtesy of The Very Little Theatre.*

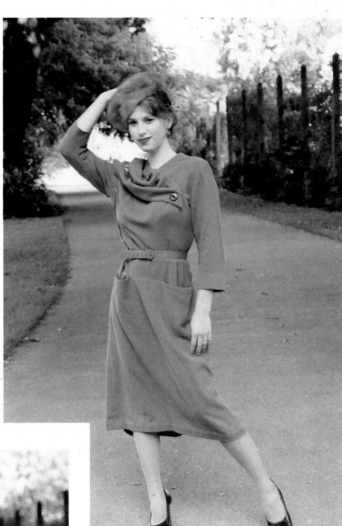

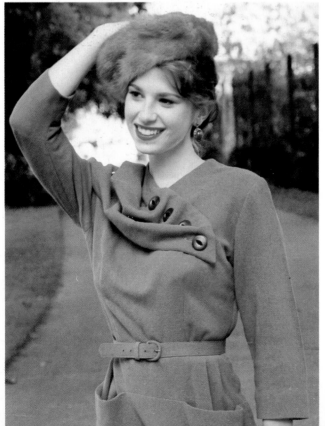

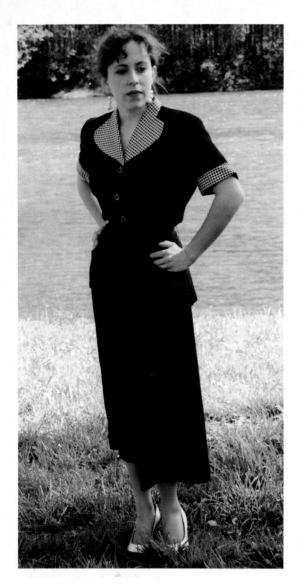

A sensible navy dress trimmed with neat checked cuffs and collar. *Courtesy of The Very Little Theatre.*

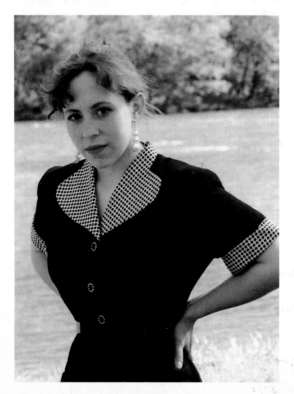

"Ever-fresh 'n' cool dotted Swiss frock, pockets and pleated sleeves frosted with dainty eyelet ruffling . . ." swooned this Tommie Austin Casuals advertisement.

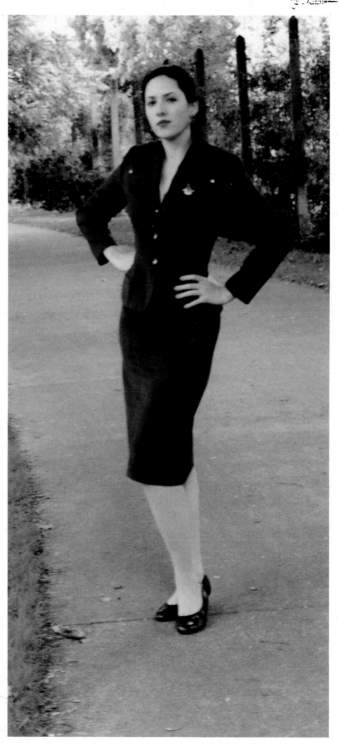

A sleek military-inspired wool suit. *Courtesy of The Very Little Theatre.*

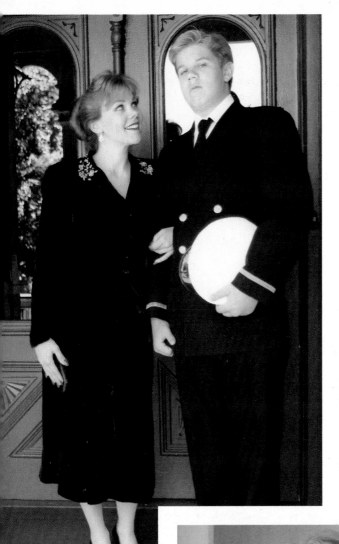

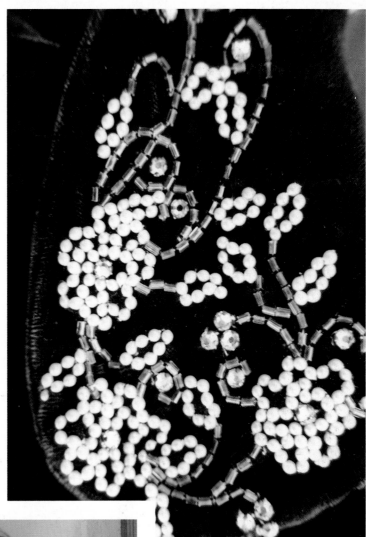

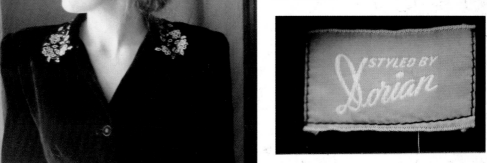

An emerald green velvet suit trimmed with beading—perfect for an evening out with a soldier on furlough. The young man wears a World War II navy ensign's uniform. *Courtesy of The Very Little Theatre.*

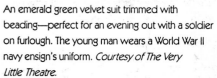

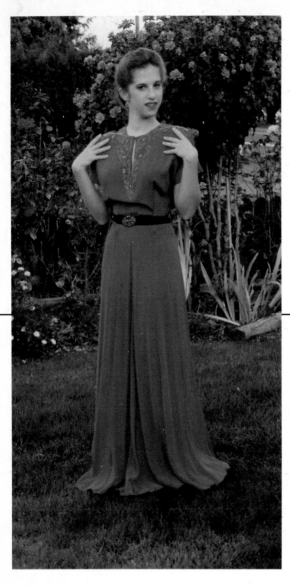

An elegant purple evening dress trimmed with cut metal beads.
Courtesy of The Very Little Theatre.

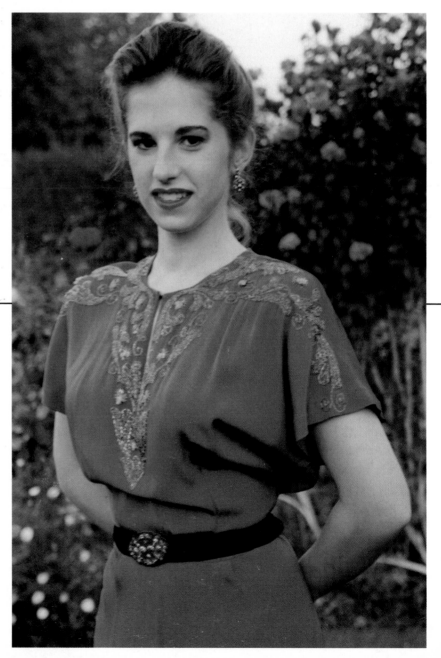

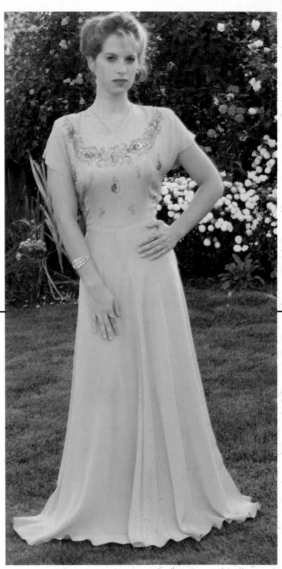

A rayon evening gown embellished with golden beads and sequins. *Courtesy of The Very Little Theatre.*

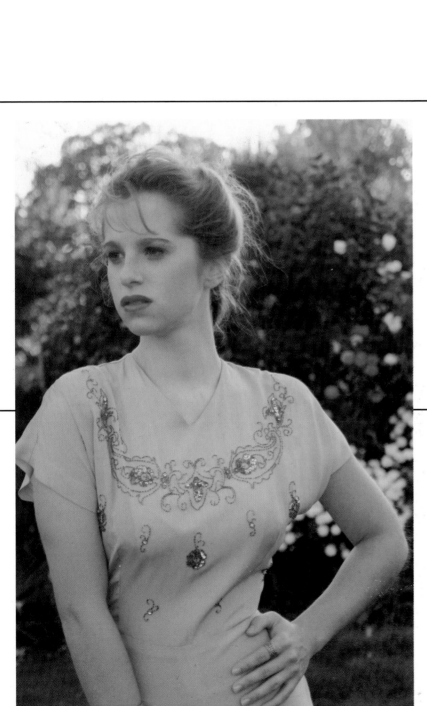

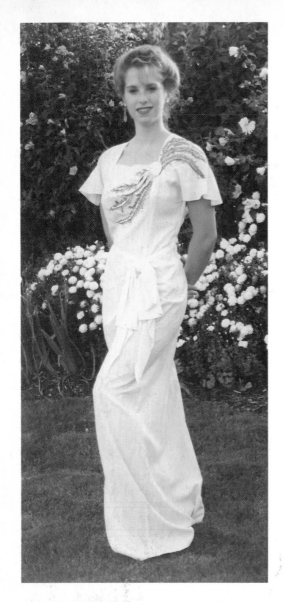

A refined white rayon evening gown trimmed with carefully-applied braid, beads, and sequins. *Courtesy of The Very Little Theatre.*

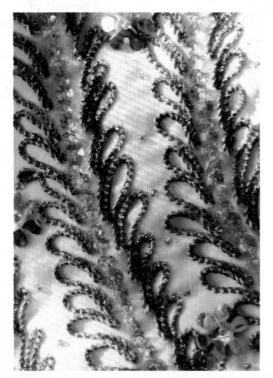

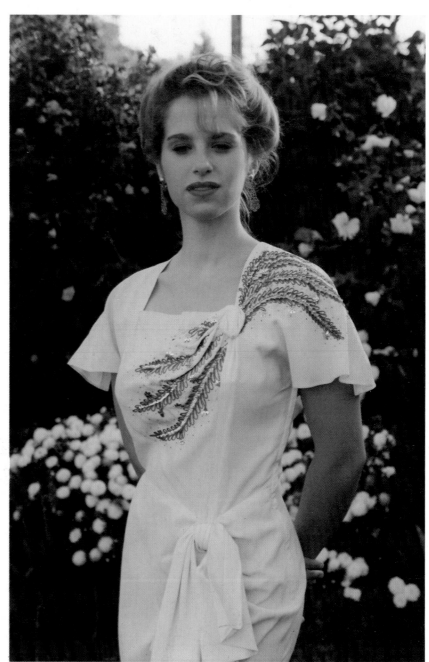

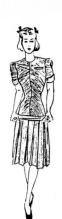

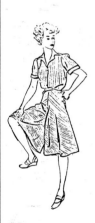

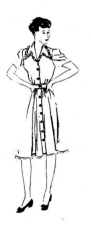

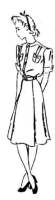

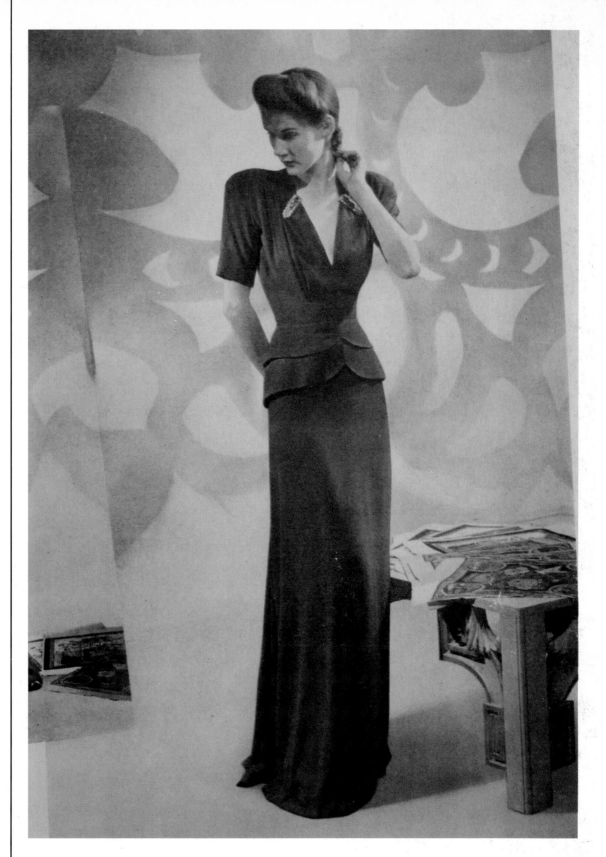

"Natural curves—your own—" this 1941 Lord & Taylor department
store advertisement touts . . . but shoulders were well-padded.
Also notice the rhinestone dress clips.

More "everyday" clothes from a 1942 issue of *Mademoiselle*: a
skirt and tunic blouse, a front-buttoned dirndl dress, culottes and a
cotton shirt, and a rayon dress.

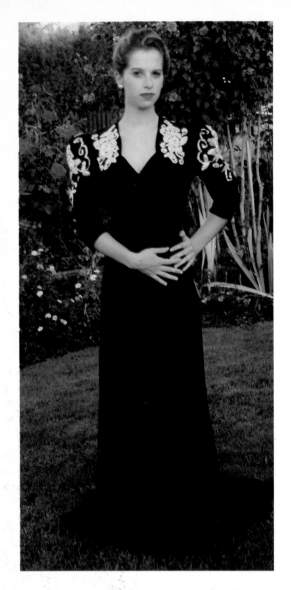

An all-forties dress of black rayon embellished with pink sequins.
Courtesy of The Very Little Theatre.

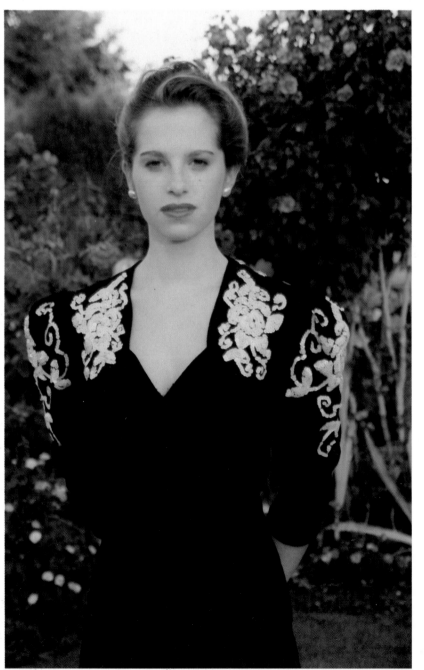

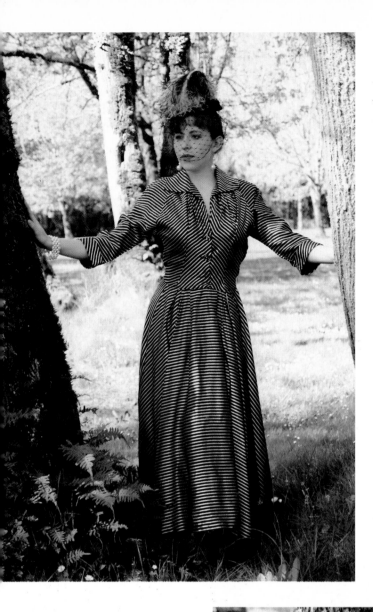

This wildly striped dress is typical of those worn late in the forties, when "The New Look" began to emerge. *Courtesy of The Very Little Theatre.*

A neo-Victorian dress with an emerald green velvet bodice closed with wooden buttons, and a skirt of striped wool, trimmed with a bustle.

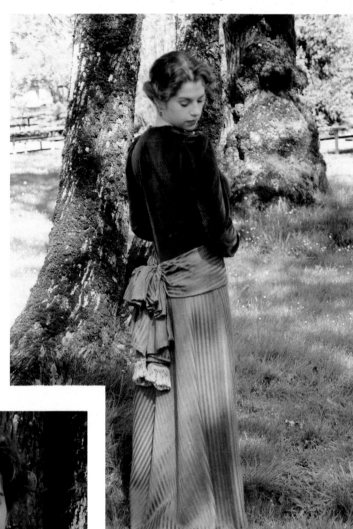

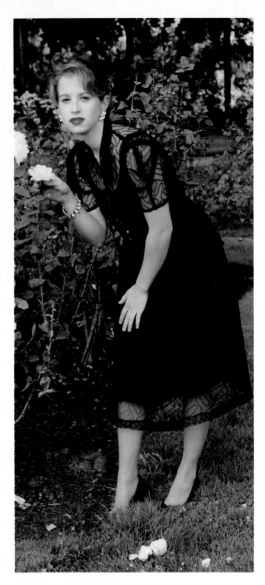

A net dress embellished with braid and rhinestone buttons.
Courtesy of The Very Little Theatre.

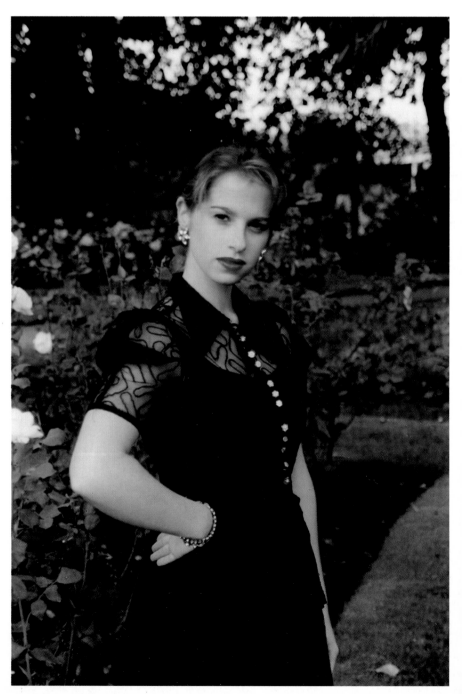

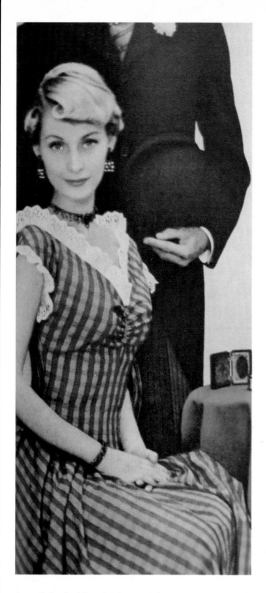

An early forties Victorian-inspired dress in taffeta gingham.

"A playtime Trio" of striped cotton, featuring shorts, skirt, and blouse, from a Dewees 1945 advertisement.

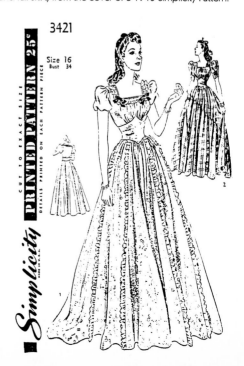

PLAYTIME TRIO
by Lynn Lester

California Candy stripes in aqua, purple and luggage on white, a HOPE SKILLMAN cotton. Sizes 12 to 18.
Blouse . . . 7.50   Shorts . . . 6.95   Skirt . . . 7.50
On mail orders please state second color choice.

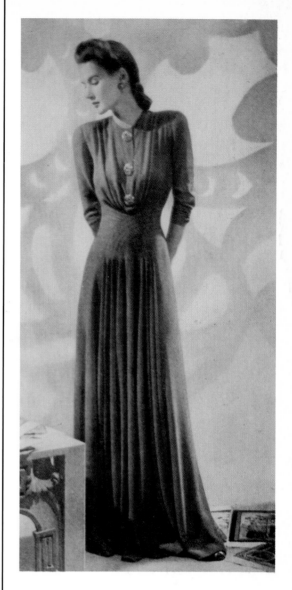

A soft, draped dress of 1941, from a Lord & Taylor department store advertisement.

A feminine, neo-Victorian dress featuring a shaped waistband and full skirt, from the cover of a 1940 Simplicity Pattern.

3421

Simplicity PRINTED PATTERN 25¢
CUT TO EXACT SIZE
DETAILS PRINTED ON EACH PATTERN PIECE

Size 16
Bust 34

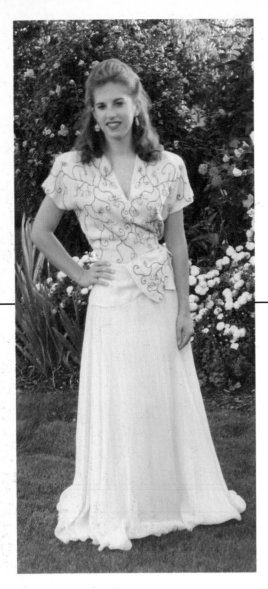

An evening gown of rayon, trimmed with exquisite beading.
Courtesy of The Very Little Theatre.

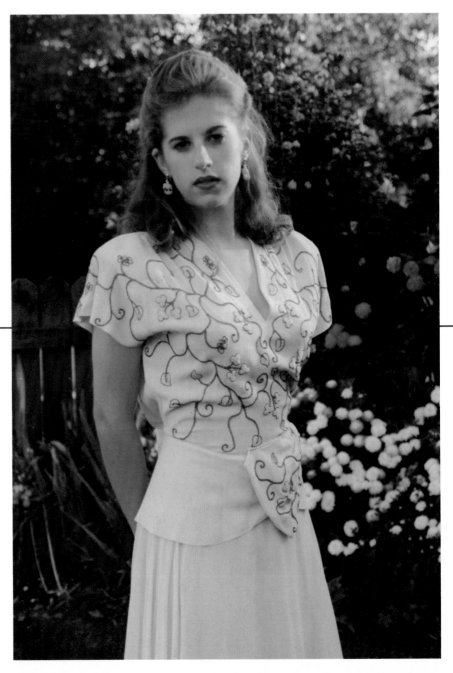

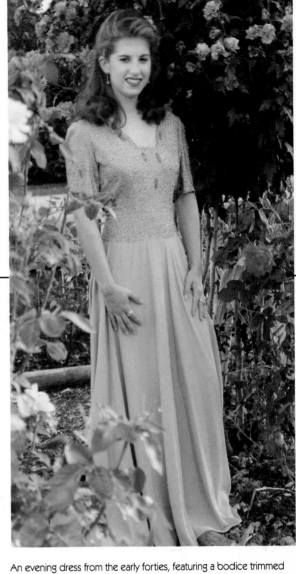

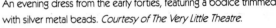

An evening dress from the early forties, featuring a bodice trimmed with silver metal beads. *Courtesy of The Very Little Theatre.*

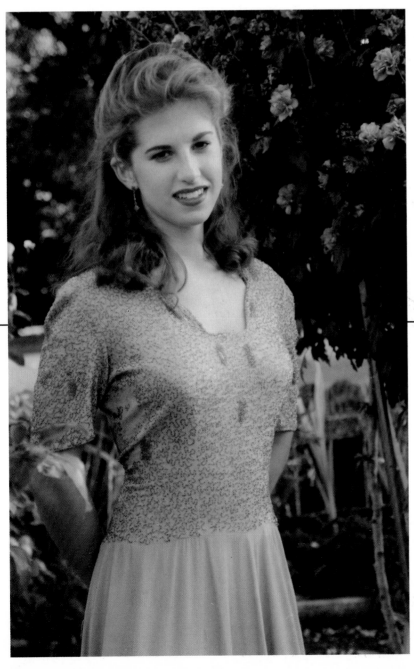

A 1947 wedding gown featuring a sweetheart neckline and cuffs shaped in elegant "V"s. The bride also kept the original McCall's pattern used to sew it. *Courtesy of Dorothy Wright.*

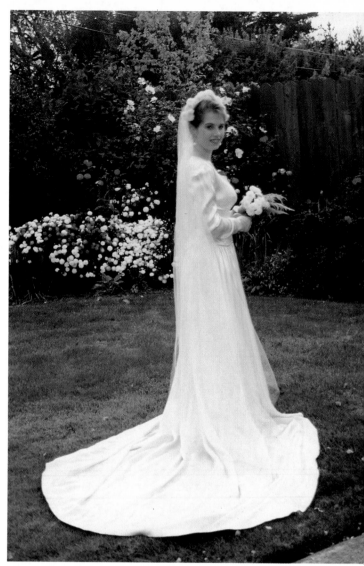

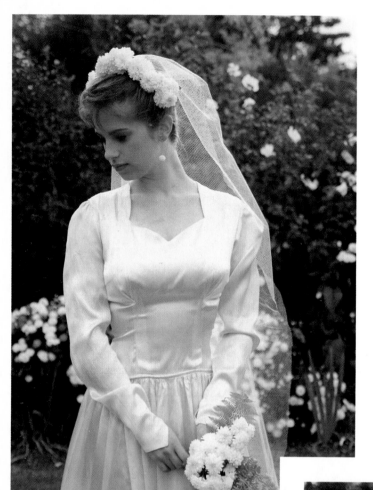

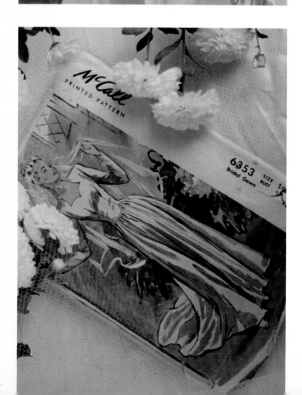

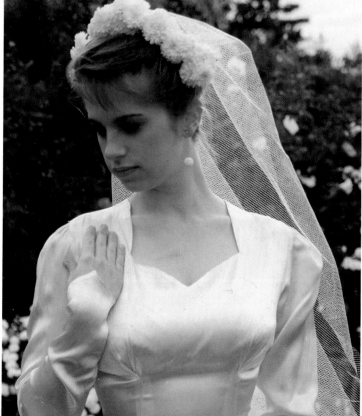

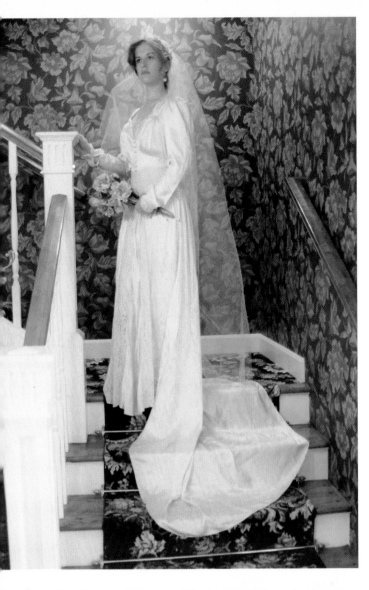

A mid–forties wedding gown with a lace waistband and a sweetheart neckline trimmed with tiny, attached, faux-pearl dress clips. *Courtesy of Marianine's Vintage Chic.*

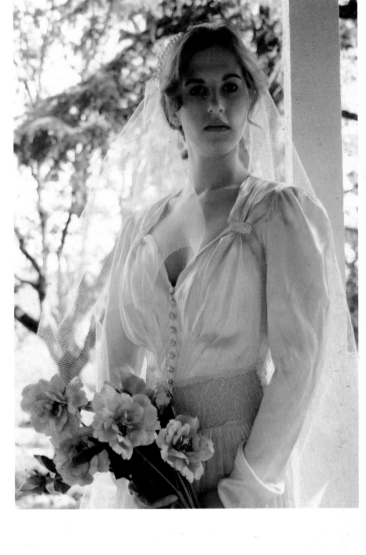

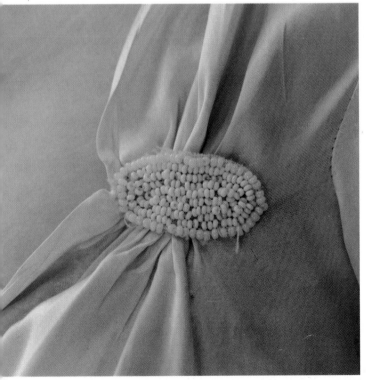

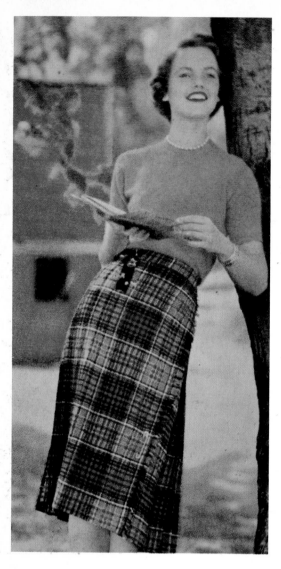

A cashmere sweater and a wrap–around–look plaid skirt: an essential part of every young ladies wardrobe, according to the August 1949 issue of *Ladies' Home Journal*.

Two full-skirted designs inspired by "the New Look" in the November 1947 *Glamour*.

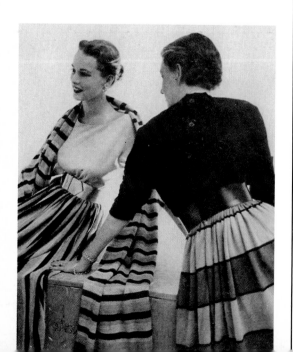

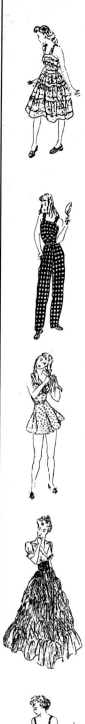

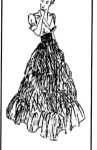

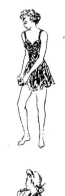

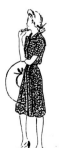

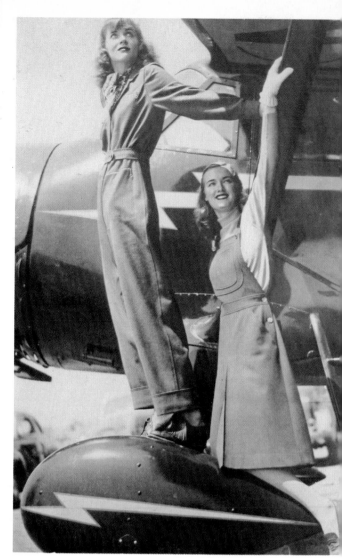

Harper's Bazaar described this Rosie-the-Riveter–style garb in 1941 as "production clothes, adapted from workmen's working clothes for the college girl to work in."

Casual wear, as seen in a 1942 issue of *Mademoiselle*: overalls, a sundress, two skirted bathing suits, a shirtwaist dress, and a full-skirted dinner dress.

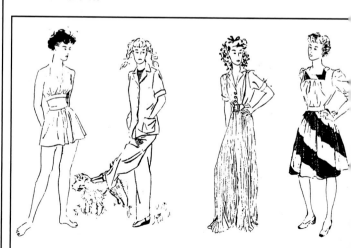

Play wear from *Mademoiselle* in 1942: a two-piece bathing suit, slacks and an over-top, and two sets of rayon skirts and blouses.

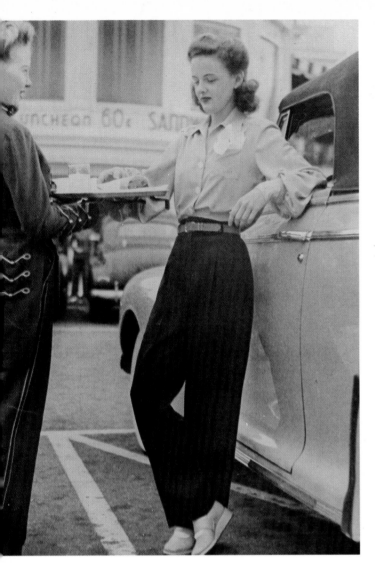

"California slacks" of rayon crepe, from a 1942 issue of *Mademoiselle*.

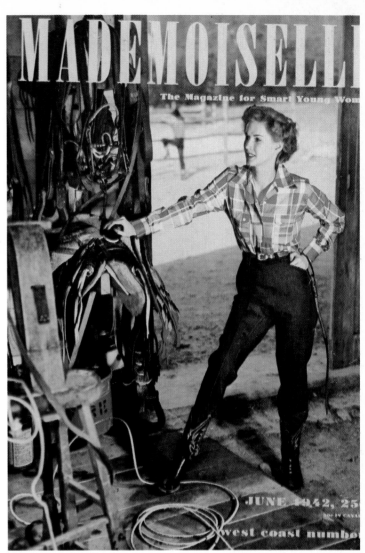

By June of 1942, *Mademoiselle* felt that pants were acceptable enough to put on their cover.

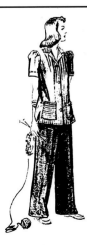

A maternity outfit featuring slacks.

In 1941, *Harper's Bazaar* featured these "frontier pants . . . tight to the leg all the way down, in heavy dark blue whipcord."

Culottes and "slim slacks," as shown in a Peck & Peck advertisement from 1942.

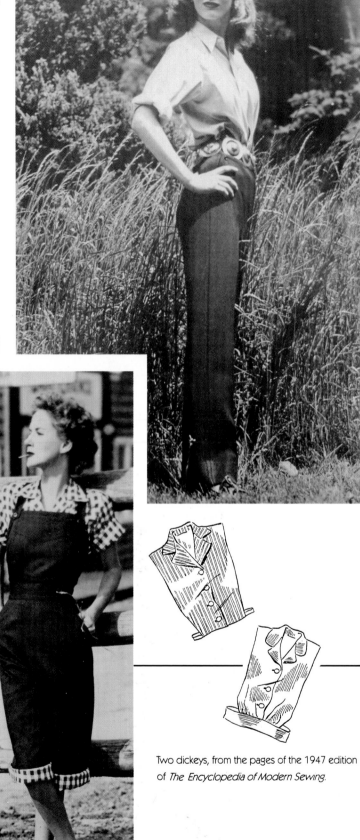

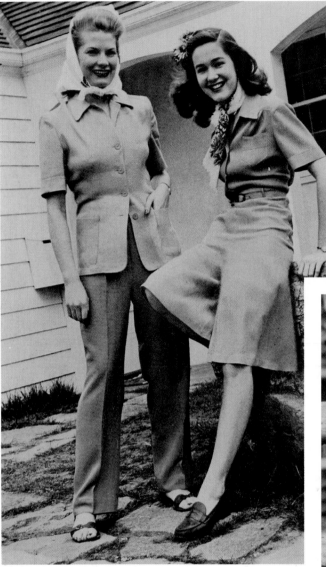

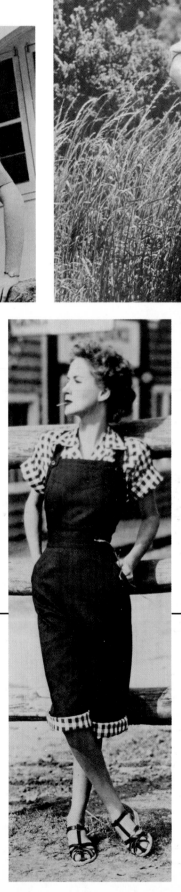

Short overalls of corded cotton, from the pages of *Mademoiselle* in 1942.

Two dickeys, from the pages of the 1947 edition of *The Encyclopedia of Modern Sewing*.

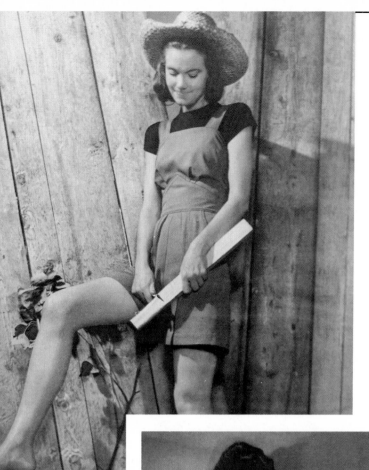

Farm-girl–style overalls from 1942.

Lounging pajamas of rayon faille with a quilted coat, from 1947.

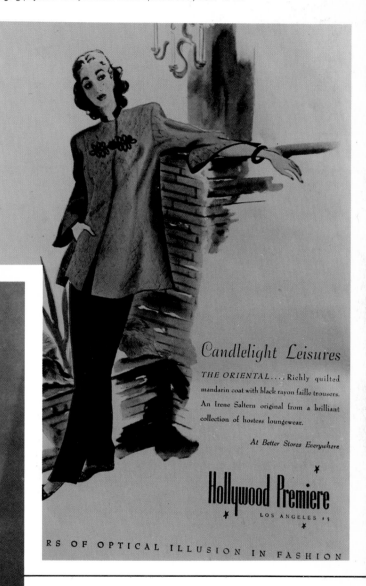

Candlelight Leisures

THE ORIENTAL.... Richly quilted mandarin coat with black rayon faille trousers. An Irene Saltern original from a brilliant collection of hostess loungewear.

At Better Stores Everywhere

Hollywood Premiere
LOS ANGELES 15

RS OF OPTICAL ILLUSION IN FASHION

A housedress, as advertised by N. Farah & Sons in 1945: "Don't bother pressing this bubble-light, washtub bright seersucker, all aflame with roses."

A piqué bikini, as featured in the June 1945 *Glamour.*

A rayon bathing suit, from the pages of *Mademoiselle.*

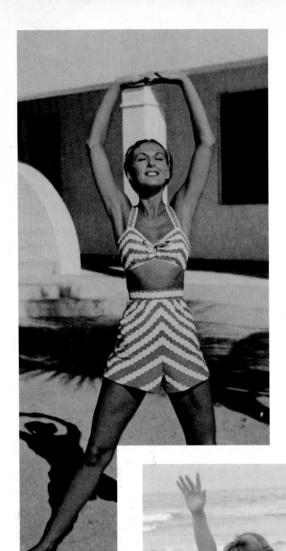

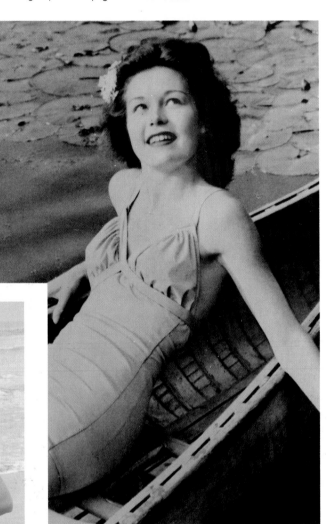

A typically forties bathing suit. *Courtesy of The Very Little Theatre.*

A bikini featured in 1949 by *Ladies' Home Journal.*

A scant bikini worn with a Mexican robozo hat, from the June 1945 issue of *Glamour.*

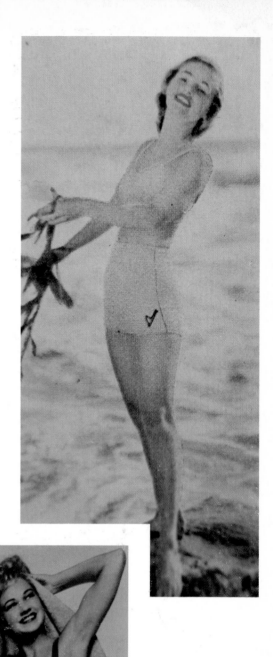

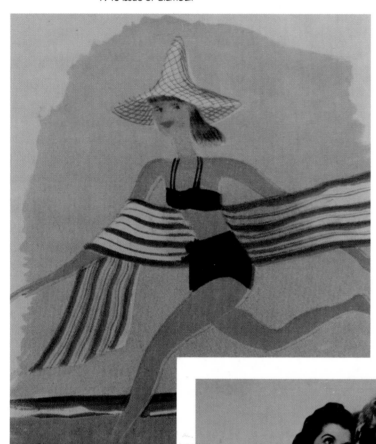

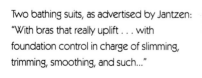

Two bathing suits, as advertised by Jantzen: "With bras that really uplift . . . with foundation control in charge of slimming, trimming, smoothing, and such..."

Typical undergarments from a Gossard advertisement: a nylon bra and girdle.

A Warner's long-line girdle from the late forties.

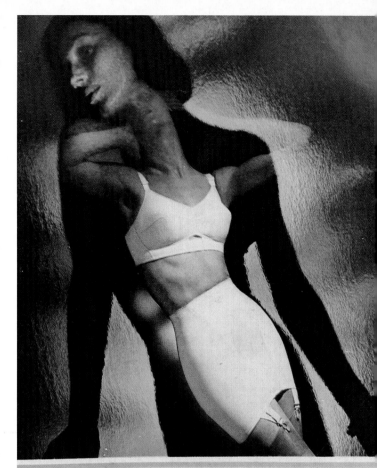

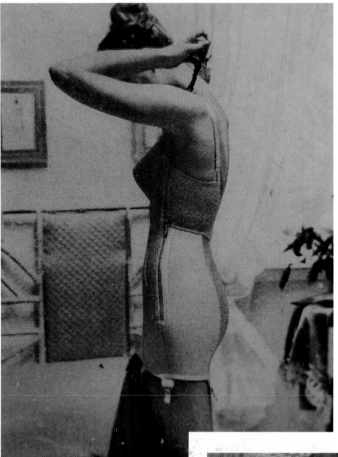

Gossar-Deb STEP-IN   Extravagantly feminine — is the word for you. Infinitesimal of waist . . . longer of mid-riff . . . higher of bosom . . . gently curving of hipline. Gossard achieved, with fastened, all Nylon step-in (satin paneled, satin leno elastic); Nylon sheer-bra.

the Gossard line of bea

A 1949 advertisement illustrating Textron brand lingerie made of the "new" tricot nylon.

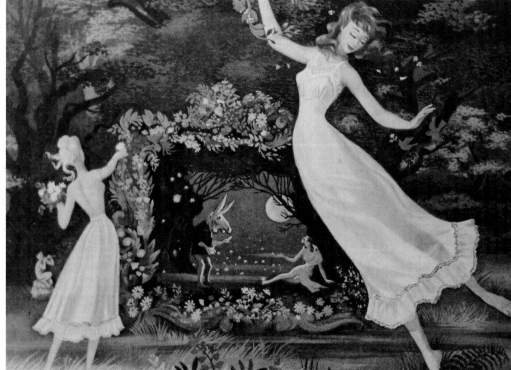

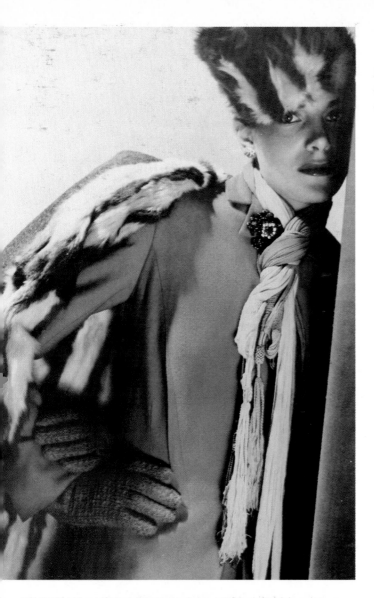

Magnificent fashion accessories, as photographed for a 1941 issue of *Harper's Bazaar*: a fur hat and stole, colorful scarves, gloves, and a costume jewelry pin.

Fashion accessories from a late 1940s Ivory Soap advertisement.

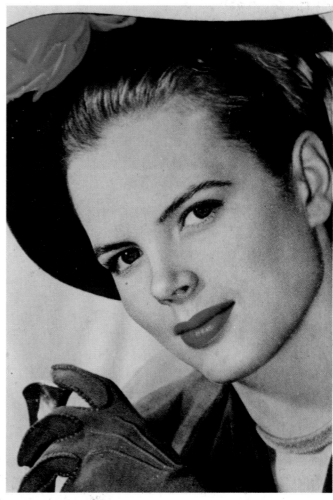

A late 1940s black satin pyramid-shaped purse embellished with beading and sequins. *Courtesy of The Very Little Theatre.*

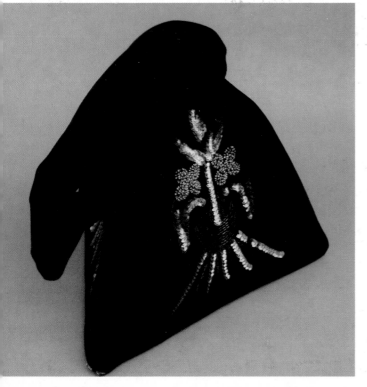

Thick-heeled pumps and platforms.

Alligator heels and handbag, advertised by the Carmo Shoe company in 1947.

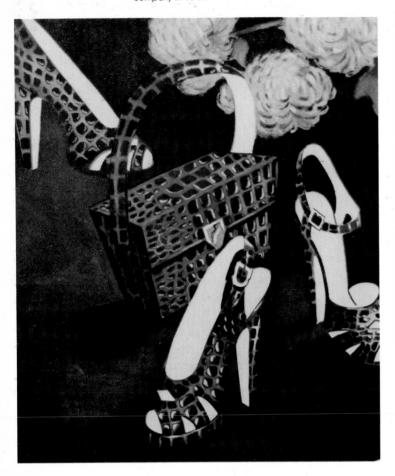

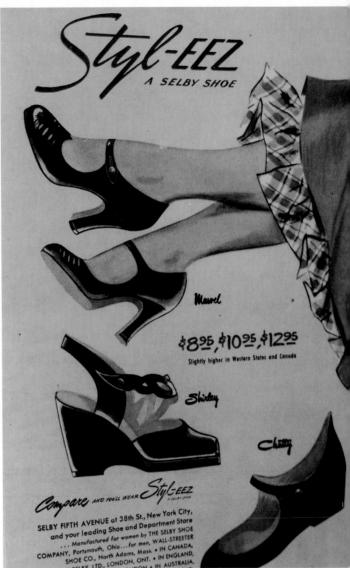

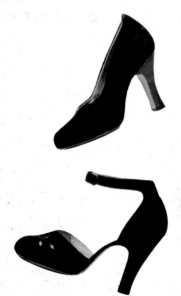

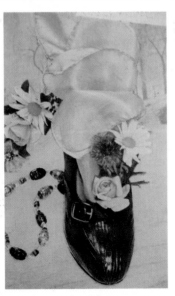

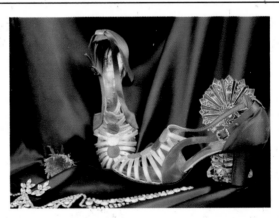

From the wide-heeled evening shoe to the leather oxford.

Rich purple evening shoes with silver, sandal-like straps. *Courtesy of The Very Little Theatre.*

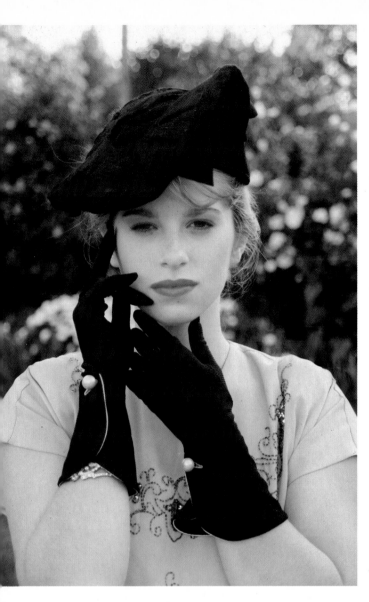

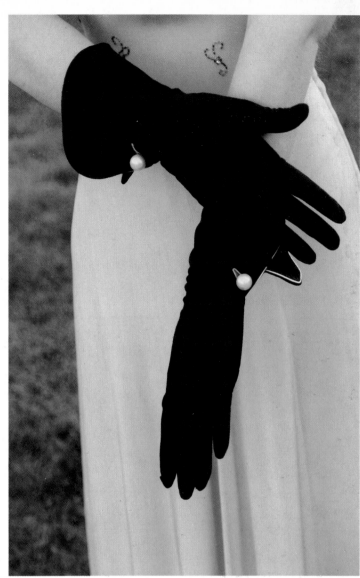

A disc-shaped felt hat. *Courtesy of The Very Little Theatre.*

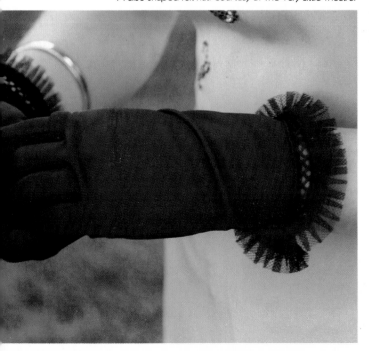

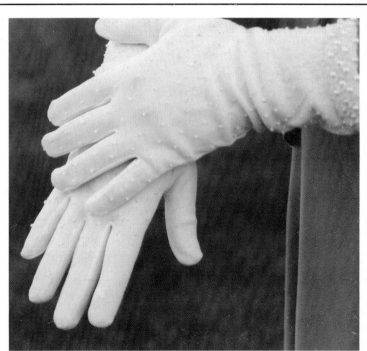

Gloves from the 1940s. *Courtesy of The Very Little Theatre.*

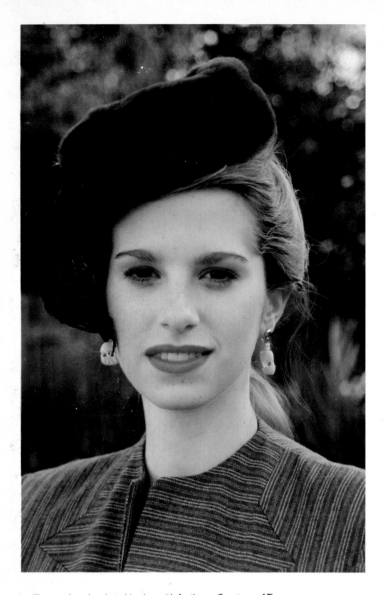

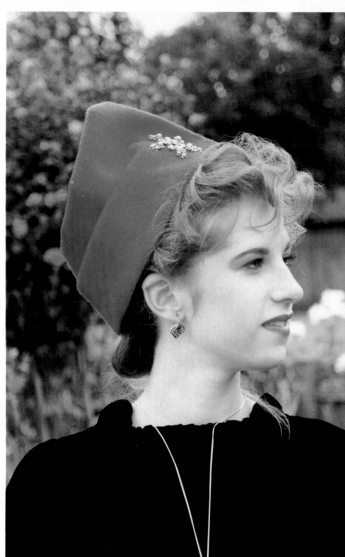

A pillbox-style velvet hat dripping with feathers. *Courtesy of The Very Little Theatre.*

Looking as if its about to take off, this bright feather hat was designed to "welcome the boys back home." *Courtesy of The Very Little Theatre.*

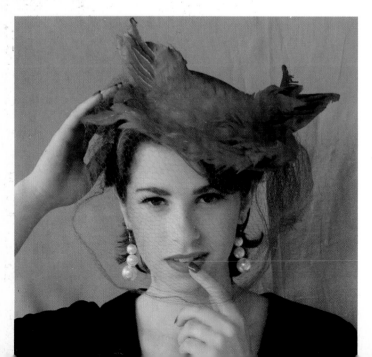

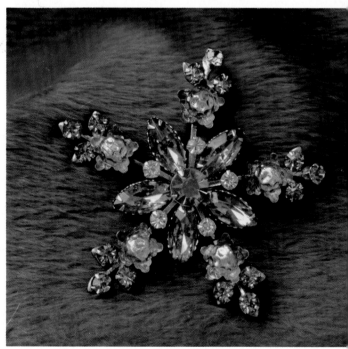

A felt, turban-like hat with an attached rhinestone snowflake. *Courtesy of The Very Little Theatre.*

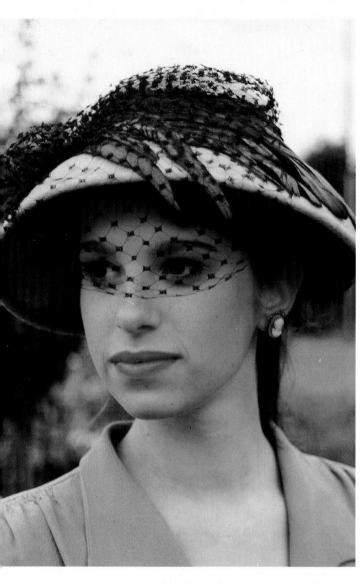

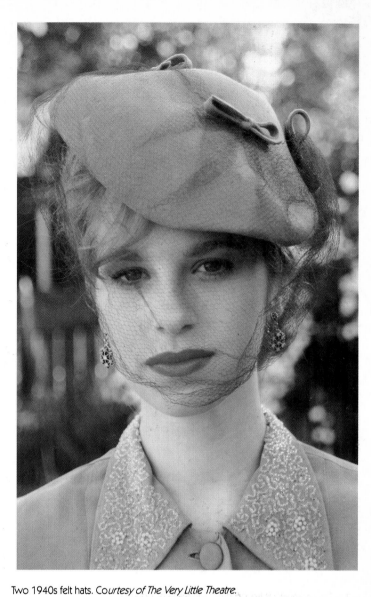

Two 1940s felt hats. *Courtesy of The Very Little Theatre.*

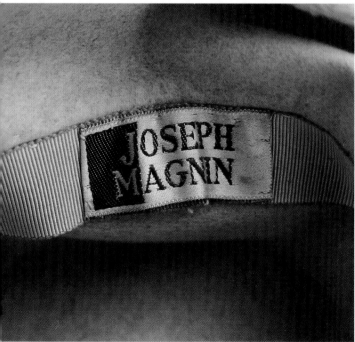

A classy Joseph Magnin felt hat. *Courtesy of The Very Little Theatre.*

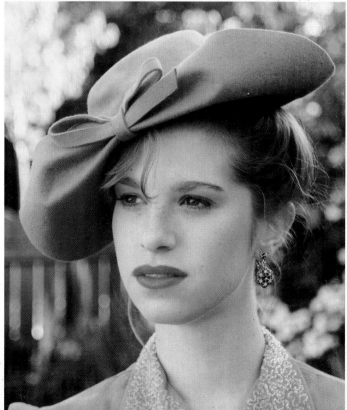

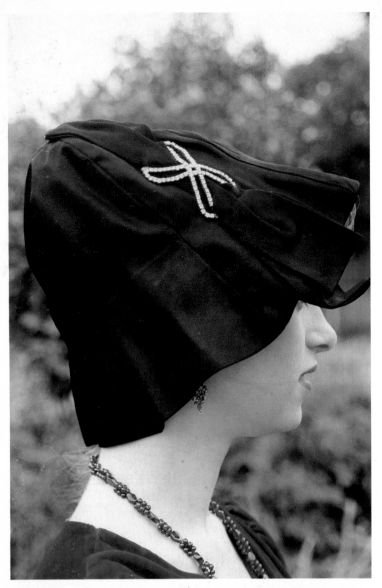

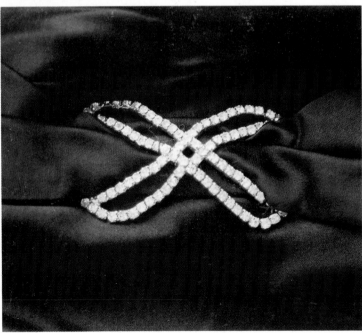

A hat, circa 1949, with an attached rhinestone clip. *Courtesy of The Very Little Theatre.*

THE "NEW LOOK"

In 1939 *Vogue* featured the return of the hourglass Victorian-style figure. But World War II interfered with this impractical, opulent style, and it wasn't until 1947 that women were able to embrace it.

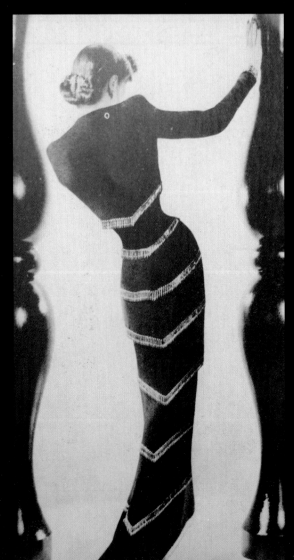

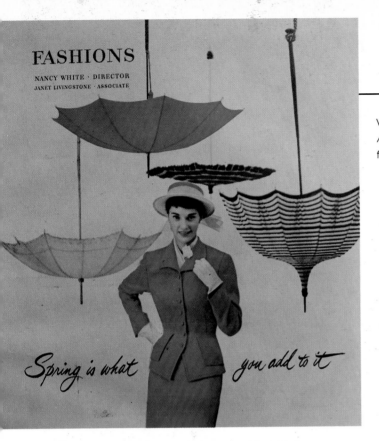

FASHIONS

NANCY WHITE · DIRECTOR
JANET LIVINGSTONE · ASSOCIATE

Spring is what *you add to it*

The New Look featured slim, figure-hugging suits and an old Victorian favorite: parasols.

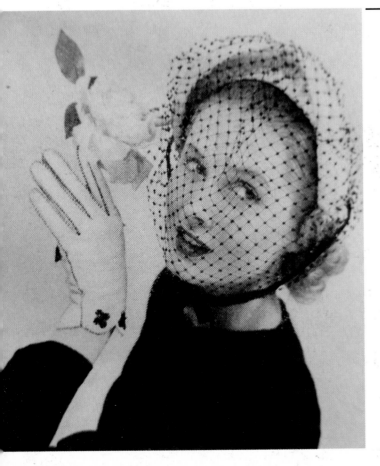

Though ladylike hats with mysterious veils had never gone out of fashion, they were essential to The New Look.

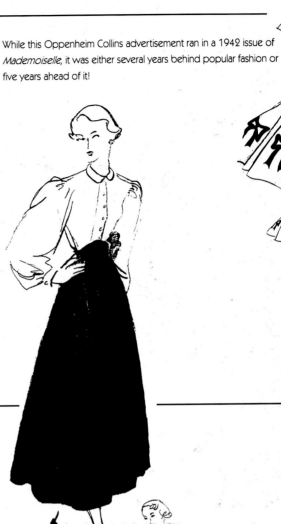

While this Oppenheim Collins advertisement ran in a 1942 issue of *Mademoiselle*, it was either several years behind popular fashion or five years ahead of it!

Early in The New Look years, turn-of-the-century Gibson Girl styles were revised and refashioned for the modern woman, as shown here in illustrations from *Glamour*.

185

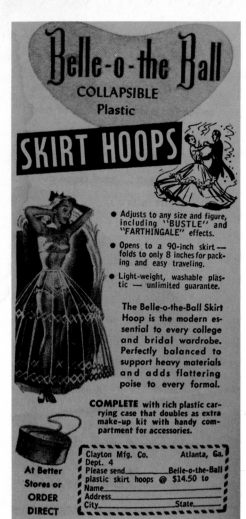
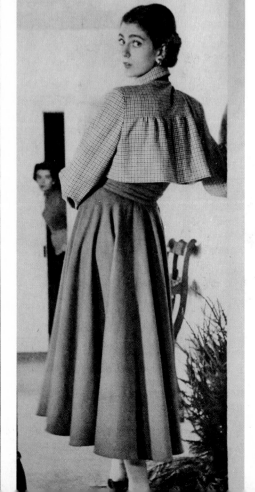

When The New Look was first introduced, Victorian-style hoopskirts were used to make skirts stand out and full.

Corsets (often called "waspies" or "waist whittlers") were also revived, as shown in this drawings from the pages of *Glamour*.

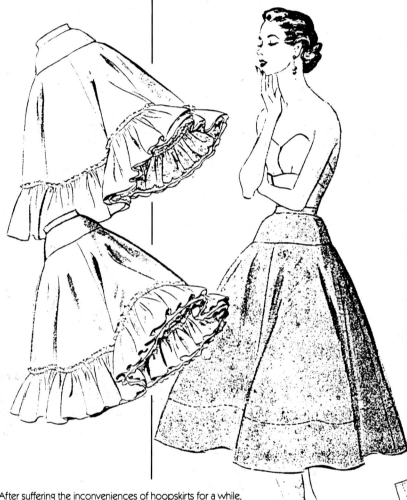

After suffering the inconveniences of hoopskirts for a while, women adopted stiffened petticoats and crinolines. For additional fullness, hip panniers could also be worn, as shown in these fashion sketches from an Advance sewing pattern.

Full skirts and full, swinging jackets were worn in 1949, as shown here from *Mademoiselle*.

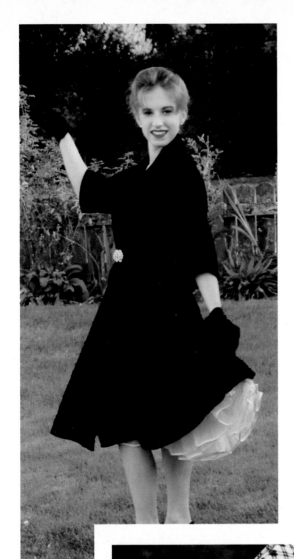

A New Look velvet coat dress worn over a pretty pink crinoline. *Dress courtesy of The Very Little Theatre.*

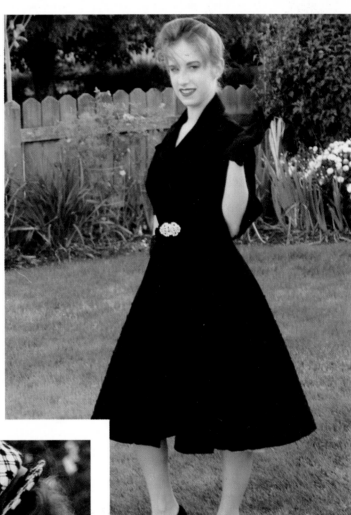

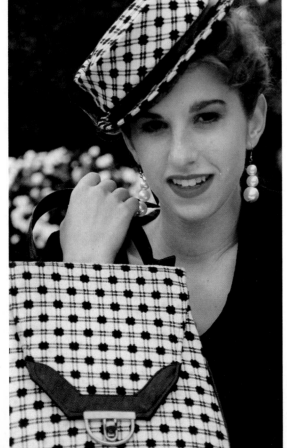

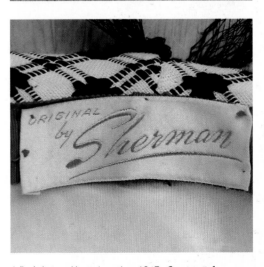

A lively hat and bag duo, circa 1947. *Courtesy of The Very Little Theatre.*

SELECTED BIBLIOGRAPHY

Among the many hundreds of books and periodicals on vintage fashions I have eagerly devoured, the following have proved particularly helpful in creating this book.

Books

Bradfield, Nancy. *Costume In Detail: 1730–1930*. Plays, Inc.: Boston, MA 1968.

Ewing, Elizabeth. *Dress and Undress*. B.T. Batsford, Ltd.: London, England 1978.

Hall, Carrie A. *From Hoopskirts To Nudity*. Caxton Printers, Ltd.: Caldwell, ID 1936.

Hall, Lee. *Common Threads*. Little, Brown, & Co.: Boston, MA 1992.

Kennett, Frances. *Collector's Book of Twentieth Century Fashion*. Granada: London, England 1983.

LaBarre, Kathleen and Kay. *Reference Book of Women's Vintage Clothing: 1920–1929*. LaBarre Books: Portland, OR 1992.

Lencêk, Lena and Gideon Bosker. *Making Waves*. Chronicle Books: San Francisco, CA 1989.

Waugh, Norah. *The Cut Of Women's Clothes*. Routeledge: New York, NY 1993.

Periodicals

Charm
Delineator, The
Fashion World: Every Woman Her Own Dressmaker
Gazette du Bon Ton
Good Housekeeping
Glamour
Harper's Bazaar
Journal des Dames et de Modes
Ladies' Home Journal
Mademoiselle
McCall's Pattern Magazine
Needlecraft
New Republic
Pictorial Review
Sears Catalog
Vanity Fair
Vogue

VALUE GUIDE

The following is intended to be a general reference for collectors and dealers who want to know the general going rates for various vintage fashion items. The listed prices come directly from dealers throughout the United States, and reflect items in excellent condition. Bear in mind that prices vary from state to state, and from region to region. Demand in your own area and current collecting trends also affect values.

When you evaluate items, every bit of damage and every flaw must be taken into consideration, and the items must be depreciated accordingly. There is no such thing as a garment in "good condition for its age"—either it *is* in good condition or it is *not*. Mint and excellent condition items from the early 1800s do exist, as do terribly torn-up garments from the 1940s.

PAGE	ITEM	VALUE						
3, 18, 63	Ensemble Dress	$300–385	33	Dress	$70–85	70	Dress	$65–80
4, 52	Sailor Dress	$25–35	34, 77	Bathing Suit	$25–35	76	Bathing Suit (set)	$80–100
6, 7, 68	Beaded Dress	$95–130	36	Dress	$20–30		Woman's alone	$40–50
9, 145	Dress	$3025–40	37	Dress	$40–65		Girl's alone	$25–35
10, 122	Evening Gown	$60–75	41	Dress	$45–70	78	Bathing Suit	$40–60
12, 83	Hat	$65–100	42	Dress	$85–100	79	Fancy Dress	
13, 143	Suit	$75–90	43	Dress	$50–70		Costume	$70–125
14, 157	Dress	$30–45	44, 45	Dress	$30–40	80	Pleated Cloche	$30–45
15, 106	Evening Gown	$65–80	45	Suit	$95–125	80	Gold-Shot Hat	$35–50
16	Sewing Patterns	$5–10 ea.	46	Dress	$35–50	81	Cloche	$15–25
16	Book	$5–12	47	Dress	$30–40	81	Needlework	
16	Notions	$1–2 each	48	Evening Dress	$30–40		Cloche	$35–45
17, 155	Dress	$45–60	49	Chiffon Dress	$20–30	82	Gold Cloche	$25–35
19, 170	Wedding Gown	$95–125	49	Woven Dress	$75–90	82	Velvet Cloche	$20–30
19, 161	Evening Gown	$760–75	50	Sailor Dress	$15–25	83	Brocade Hat	$20–35
19, 148	Suit	$35–50	50	Lace Dress	$75–90	84	Evening Cap	$30–40
20, 71	Beaded Blouse	$65–80	51	Dress	$25–35	84	Headdress	$180–200
20, 64	Beaded Dress	$150–250	53	Border Print Dress	$35–45	85	Beaded Comb	$45–60
20, 138	Blue Beaded		53	Chiffon Dress	$35–45	85	Faux Tortoise	
	Dress	$180–250	54	Dress	$70–90		Shell Comb	$25–35
21, 114	Dress	$70–85	55	Chiffon Dress	$30–45	88	Reticule	$75–85
21, 83	Crocheted		55	Beaded Dress	$35–50	88	Beaded Purse	$75–90
	Boudoir Cap	$10–20	56	Velvet Dress	$35–50	88	Brocade Purse	$25–35
21, 82	Silk Boudoir Cap	$15–20	56	Coat Dress	$15–25	88, 89	Metal Frame Bag	$45–60
22, 26, 171	Wedding Gown	$100–200	57	Chiffon Dress	$30–40	89	Silk Reticule	$35–50
24, 108	Evening Gown	$90–100	57	Lace Dress	$85–130	89	Makeup Purse	$60–80
24, 102	Dress	$65–75	58	Dress	$80–95	91	Satin Coat	$50–65
25, 176	Bathing Suit	$25–35	59	Dress	$70–90	91	Cape	$55–70
25, 135	Hat	$45–65	60	Dress	$60–75	92	Coat	$50–65
25, 169	Beaded Dress	$50–65	61	Dress	$50–65	93	Coat	$70–85
26, 38	Hat	$35–45	62	Dress	$60–75	94	Coat	$75–90
26, 38	Dress	$25–35	65	Dress	$150–250	95	Shawl	$25–35
27, 130	Dress	$65–80	66	Dress	$65–80	96	Shawl	$65–75
30, 31	Evening Gown	$150–200	67	Dress	$70–90	97	Shawl	$25–35
31	Dress	$75–95	69	Dress	$900–1,000	98	Silk Shoes	$60–70

98	Brocade Shoes	$30–45	128	Black Dress	$70–80	159	Suit	$70–85
99	Shoes	$45–60	128	Blue Dress	$70–95	158	Ensign's Uniform	$120-130
100, 123	Evening Gown	$85–100	129	Ruched Velvet		160	Dress	$65–75
103	Dress	$45–65		Dress	$40–55	162	Dress	$80–100
105	Net Dress	$45–65	129	Blue Velvet Dress	$70–95	164	Dress	$70–80
107	Dress	$45–65	130	Net Dress	$75–85	165	Striped Dress	$25–35
108	Dress	$95–120	134	Bathing Suit	$20–30	165	Bustle Dress	$65–85
109	Print Dress	$15–25	134	Velvet Hat	$15–25	166	Dress	$65–75
109	Dress	$15–25	134	Eugenie Hat	$35–45	168	Dress	$80–100
110,111	Dress	$70–90	135	Plumed Eugenie		179	Purse	$15–25
112	Satin Dress	$40–60		Hat	$50–60	180	Shoes	$25–35
112, 113	Crepe Dress	$35–45	135	Printed Shoes	$30–40	181	Hat	$15–20
114	Plaid Dress	$25–30	135	Iridescent Shoes	$15–25	181	Gloves	$5–15 each
115	Dress	$50–65	139	Dress	$25–30	182	Velvet Pillbox	$8–15
116	Dress	$30–40	140	Dress	$25–35	182	Felt & Rhinestone	
117	Dress	$20–25	143	Day Suit	$40–65		Hat	$10–15
118	Organdy Dress	$70–90	144	Suit	$65–80	182	Feather Hat	$30–45
118	Pleated Dress	$30–40	146	Polka-Dot		183	J. Magnin Hat	$10–25
119	Dress	$60–85		Jacket	$25–30	183	Felt Beret	$8–20
120	Fringed Dress	$40–50	146	Suit	$65–80	183	Hat	$10–25
120	Bridesmaid's		150	Suit	$35–40	184	Hat	$10–20
	Dress	$25–35	152	Dress	$70–80	197	Hat & Purse (set)	$30–40
121	Dress	$30–40	153	Dress	$55–65		Hat alone	$8–10
124	Dress	$75–90	154	Suit	$45–60		Purse alone	$10–15
125	Dress	$50–65	156	Dress	$65–80	187	Dress	$70–85
126	Dress	$40–60	157	Suit	$70–85	187	Crinoline	$25–40
127	Dress	$100–120	158	Dress	$25–35			

MODELING CREDITS

Anna Kristine Crivello: 4, 52, 76

Clinton McKay Crivello: 159

Lisa Ann Crivello: 10, 15, 20 (TR), 25 (TL), 31 (R), 34, 70, 76, 77, 78, 100, 105, 106, 115, 122, 123, 126, 129 (R), 134 (TL), 138, 152, 159, 176

Darcie Jones: 3, 12, 17, 18, 19 (BR), 21, 22, 25 (B), 26 (C, BL), 33, 41, 43, 45 (TR, B), 47, 50 (TL), 53 (B), 54, 56 (L), 59, 61, 62, 63, 66, 67, 82 (BL), 83 (TR, BR), 92, 103, 109 (TR), 110, 111, 118 (TL), 119, 128 (TL, B), 134 (TR), 143 (R), 144, 148, 155, 157 (TL), 160, 168, 169, 171, 182 (TR), 187

Joslin Jones: 42, 49 (TR), 57 (R), 82 (TL), 83 (TL), 91 (B), 94, 108 (TR), 114 (B), 118 (TR, B), 120 (TR, BR), 121, 134 (B), 135 (B), 146 (TL), 150, 158 (TL, B), 165 (TL)

Stephanie Jones: 6, 9, 13, 14, 19 (C, TR), 20 (C, L), 21 (T), 24 (L), 25 (TR), 30, 31 (L), 36, 44, 45 (TL), 46, 48, 49 (TL, B), 50 (TR), 51, 53 (TL, TR), 55, 56 (R), 57 (L), 58, 60, 64, 65, 68, 69, 71, 79, 82 (TR, BR), 84 (L), 91 (T), 93, 96, 97, 107, 108 (TL, B), 109 (TL), 112 (TL), 113, 114 (TL), 117, 124, 125, 127, 129 (L), 130 (B), 135 (T), 139, 143 (L), 145, 146 (TR, B), 153, 154, 157 (TR, B), 161, 162, 164, 165 (TR, B), 166, 170, 181, 182 (TL, BL), 183, 184

Alicia Lafayette: 26 (TL), 37, 38, 80, 81, 116

Virginia Speckman: 24 (R), 27, 84 (R), 95, 102, 112 (TL, B), 120 (TL, BL), 128 (R), 130 (TL), 140, 156, 158 (L)

INDEX